Tank Top
Arms

Bikini Belly

Boy Shorts
Bottom

FOR EVERY WOMAN,
YOUNG AND OLD,
WHO BELIEVES IN HERSELF AND
IN THE WISDOM IN HER HEART.

CONTENTS

ACKNOWLEDGMENTS

To my family: You have given more of yourselves than imaginable, and I thank you for your tremendous amount of love, support, and encouragement. Thank you to:

Joseph Amuial, my husband, for all that you are and all that you do—you are the best man I know. And to our daughters: Ema and Mia, you are my inspiration and the brightest souls.

My loving parents, David and Sira Lessig. Mom, thanks for talking the talk and walking the walk of health and fitness and keeping me on that path with you—you continue to be an inspiration. Dad, through word and example, you've helped me achieve by teaching me the value of hard work and dedication.

Jacob and Terri Amuial, my loving father- and mother-in-law, for your always-present abundant love and support.

My most wonderful grandparents, William R. Lessig Jr. and June Lessig, and Anne Gilbert. Alisa, Brad, Jake, and Josie, I love you. And my faraway family: Mummo, Katja, Tiina, and Nico: for always sending your love and positive thoughts. Katja: an extra special thank-you for the beloved friend you are to me.

A very special thank-you to two treasured friends, Bianca Diaz, a.k.a. Angel, and Jacqueline Dutra: You are always in my heart, now and through lifetimes.

To all my wonderful clients and friends who have placed their belief and trust in me, thank you for allowing me to help you reach your highest goals: Elizabeth Pritchard, Andi Greenwald, Sarah, Barbara F., Jim, Matt, Janice, Dan, and the many students who have crossed my path.

Thank you to my trainers and staff at Great Neck Personal Trainer: I am proud of my team; you guys are the best trainers in Virginia Beach!

Many, many, many thanks to Andrea Ambandos, the all-time best producer and coolest person I am honored to have worked with and know.

Annmarie Gatti, thank you for your genuine support and all your help.

Thank you to my lawyer, Scott Seymour, of Kaufman & Canoles: An artist has true freedom of creativity when she has people like you on her side.

A very heartfelt thank-you to all the people at Rodale who have worked hard to make this happen, are exceptional at what they do, and have made it such an enjoyable project to take on. Amy Super: It's been a dream to do this. A special thank-you to you in the first place for getting it all started. Julia VanTine-Reichardt: You are amazing at what you do, and I thank you for all your guidance and for making it fun! Susan Eugster: Thanks for extending your help and care to my family as well. Mitch Mandel and Troy Schneider: Thanks for a great shoot—the most relaxed and enjoyable one, and thanks for all the great music to keep the energy going! Adrianne Beardem: A million crunches couldn't work my abs half as much as your jokes— thanks for all the laughs (and for your phenomenal work)! Marc Sirinsky: Thanks for the many ways you helped! Lois Hazel: Thank you for your hard work and dedication to keeping the ball rolling.

Last, a most special thank-you to an amazing woman who continues to live within me . . . my grandmother, Miriam Reiniger Lessig. You are my Angel.

INTRODUCTION

You've tried to slim down and shape up—more than once, perhaps. But something has always foiled your intentions: No time to work out. No money for a gym membership. No results, despite your best efforts. No motivation—the biggest obstacle of all.

This time, things will be different. And "this time" starts today.

In just 4 short weeks, a leaner, more sculpted body can be yours. As a professional athlete, personal trainer, fitness model, and TV fitness personality, I can make such promises. In person, with my fitness videos, and in magazine and TV workouts, I've helped countless women achieve the fit, lean bodies they always wanted.

Now it's your turn. My program can take your body to a new level of grace, strength, and fitness. You'll slip into clothing you've longed to wear: cute bikinis with boy shorts bottoms that reveal a leaner lower body. Tank tops that expose toned arms and sculpted shoulders. Low-rise jeans that show off a taut, toned belly.

"This time" starts with strength training, a critical component of a balanced fitness program. Lifting weights builds firm, shapely, feminine muscle that burns 10 times more calories than its weight in fat.

Here's what you can expect from my program.

A FITNESS "PRESCRIPTION" FOR EVERY FITNESS LEVEL. Whether you're an absolute beginner or looking for new and challenging routines, I've got you covered with Novice, Skilled, and Master exercises and workouts. No matter where you're starting from, in 30 days you'll see significant fat loss and dramatic improvements in your strength, flexibility, and balance.

FLEXIBILITY. You can do my program at home with minimal equipment or at the gym. As a bonus, with each exercise I offer variations for both home and gym workouts.

FRESH MOVES. If you're tired of the same old routines, you've come to the right place. I give traditional strength-training exercises a twist, adding moves from yoga, dance, gymnastics, and Pilates. I round out the program with flexibility training and cardiovascular exercise for an effective, time-efficient workout.

BUILT-IN MOTIVATION. As an athlete, I learned the value of visualization and other mental training tools in achieving peak performance. Peak performance yields peak results: a strong, lean, fit body. Incorporate one or all of the tools presented on these pages into your program, and watch as your motivation—and the result—reaches the next level.

CUTTING-EDGE TRAINING PRINCIPLES. Ripped abs aren't worth much if you wrench your back lifting the laundry basket. That's why I've based my program on the principles of *functional training*. Unlike traditional strength training, which works individual muscles in isolation, functional-training exercises work multiple

DETERMINING YOUR FITNESS LEVEL

To ensure your success, it's important to start with the moves and program that match your current fitness level: Novice, Skilled, or Master. These guidelines can help. Note: If you have heart disease, diabetes, or any other chronic health condition, or are more than 50 pounds over your ideal weight, talk to your doctor before you begin this or any fitness program. Also, if a particular exercise or workout feels too hard, replace it with a less-demanding move or program, then attempt it again as you gain strength, flexibility, and balance. Remember: Your body knows best. If it doesn't feel good, don't do it.

Start with the Novice Program if you:

❖ are completely new to exercise

❖ have not exercised in 6 months or more

Start with the Skilled Program if you:

❖ have been exercising for 6 months or more

❖ can perform the Novice Program exercises in this book with correct technique

Start with the Master Program if you:

❖ have been exercising for 1 year or more

❖ can perform the Novice Program and Skilled Program exercises in this book with correct technique

❖ are injury free

MIND TOOL: AFFIRMATIONS

Affirmations are statements used to boost self-esteem. They are worded in a positive rather than a negative way and are grounded in the present rather than the future. An example of a positive affirmation for weight loss is "I am losing weight and getting fit." Repeat these affirmations enough and your subconscious will come to believe them, replacing a negative interior dialogue with a more positive one. Affirmations don't work their magic right away, however. You need to repeat them dozens of times a day, aloud and to yourself, writing them, reading them, letting them sink inside until they reach the deepest part of your being. Other examples of affirmations include:

- ❖ "I have strong, flexible, lean muscles."
- ❖ "My body is fit and beautiful."
- ❖ "I love my strong, healthy, fit body."

These are only examples. Feel free to make up your own affirmations. "Personalized" affirmations are much more powerful.

muscles and joints together in ways that mimic everyday activities. In my program, you don't just "lift weights." You use free weights in specific ways that build flexibility, balance, and coordination as well as strength. Read on to learn more about this unique style of training.

THE BENEFITS OF FUNCTIONAL TRAINING

When you hold a squirming toddler, bend to retrieve a pair of shoes in your closet, or hang a picture on your living-room wall, your body isn't using one muscle in isolation but many muscles that work *together*.

That's why functional-training exercises mimic the movements of everyday life: bending and reaching as you put away groceries, washing your dog in the tub, moving the couch away from the wall to vacuum behind it. That's because the exercises force your *core*—the muscles of your groin, upper back, and chest, as well as your abdomen—to work harder and get stronger. Functional training also focuses on *joint integrity*, which is the ability to maintain posture, control motion, and keep your balance. The benefits: The demands of everyday life become a lot easier, and you're less likely to injure yourself stooping to pick up your overflowing laundry basket.

Don't let the name intimidate you. If you've ever performed crunches on a stability ball, you're already familiar with functional training. This move doesn't just "work your abs," it calls upon other muscles in your pelvis, back, and hips to maintain your balance. This increased effort builds more muscle, and the more muscle you have, the more calories you burn.

Which brings us back to my promise: My program will help you shed excess body fat and sculpt sleek, feminine muscle. But it will also make those muscles *functional*, thereby improving your quality of life.

HOW TO USE THIS BOOK

I know you're eager to plunge into the program, but give me a second to explain how you should proceed. In The Cardio Equation (see page 7), you'll discover how and why cardiovascular exercise accelerates fat loss, as well as the particulars of my cardio workout—how much, how often, and how to perform it safely and effectively.

MIND TOOL: POSITIVE SELF-TALK

Psychologists believe that our self-talk—the words we use when we talk to ourselves—influences our self-esteem, outlook, performance, and relationships. And it definitely can affect our health, determining, for example, how easily we replace unhealthy behaviors with healthy ones. *Positive self-talk* is internal dialogue that is loving and encouraging, rather than negative and harsh. It's talking to yourself the way you would to a 4-year-old trying to stack blocks or an 8-year-old trying to ride a two-wheeler for the first time. To try positive self-talk on yourself, imagine a kind, supportive voice—the voice of a grandparent, coach, favorite teacher, or friend—saying things like "You can do it—I know you can" or "You did it! I'm so proud of you!"

Just as important as encouraging yourself to do more or try harder is giving yourself a rest when you need one. Remind yourself that everyone needs a break occasionally: "I may not have it in me to do 1 more set of this exercise today, but I have tried my best, and I feel good about that!"

(There's even a cool treadmill-walking workout to try.) In Stretch Yourself (see page 19), I reveal the benefits of stretching and introduce you to the stretches that I recommend you do after each exercise.

Parts 1 through 3 present the exercises. Part 1, Tank Top Arms, focuses on moves that firm and tone the upper body, including the shoulders, arms, and back. Part 2, Bikini Belly, introduces moves that strengthen your core musculature and flatten your belly. Part 3, Boy Shorts Bottom, presents moves that slim and sculpt the lower body, including the legs, hips, and butt.

I've divided each part by fitness level. In the Tank Top Arms part, for example, you'll find moves specifically selected for your fitness level: Novice, Skilled, and Master. Determine your fitness level (see the sidebar on page 2), then perform the moves in that section.

Part 4, Putting It All Together, presents the workouts I designed to meet the unique needs and challenges of each fitness level. The Novice Level (see page 213) trains the entire body. The Skilled Level (see page 225) alternates between upper and lower body workouts. The Master Level (see page 241) focuses on perfecting specific body parts.

In the Appendix, Staying Lean for Life: Nutrition Principles and Practice (see page 263), you'll find practical advice for eating for weight loss and training—the same advice that I follow. (My diet is far from perfect, and I don't expect yours to be, either!) I've also included training logs (page 281) that allow you to monitor your progress.

❖

THE CARDIO EQUATION

A "fit" body doesn't just look good on the outside—it's healthy on the inside, too. That's why cardiovascular exercise, or *cardio*, is a vital component of a balanced fitness program. Engaging in regular, moderate-intensity cardio does more than help you slide into skinny jeans. It also strengthens your heart and lungs, helps reduce the risk of developing chronic conditions such as high blood cholesterol levels and cancer, and boosts your mental and emotional well-being.

When it comes to cardio, the preferred type is . . . the type you enjoy. There is no "best" cardio, because what counts is not what you do but the effort you put into it. Any activity that raises your heart rate for at least 20 minutes fits the bill. Fortunately, cardio comes in almost as many varieties as ice cream. There are the vanilla, chocolate, and strawberry of cardio—walking, jogging, and aerobics—but for more exotic "flavors," check out the table on page 12. You may be surprised by the wide variety of activities that constitute "cardio." You may have so much fun, you'll forget that you're working out!

Still, there are a few things you need to know before you lace up your sneakers. Especially if you're a beginner, you should consider this chapter a primer on aerobic exercise—Cardio 101, if you will.

CARDIO'S BIG THREE

Safe and effective aerobic-training guidelines include recommendations on frequency, intensity, and time (FIT). Understanding these components will make your cardio workout as safe and effective as possible.

FREQUENCY: *Frequency* refers to how often you exercise. Most fitness experts, myself included, recommend cardio at least 3 times a week—and 4 or 5 days is better.

INTENSITY: Experts categorize the *intensity* of physical activity as low, moderate, or high based on the amount of effort you expend. Performing cardio at the proper intensity level *for you* can significantly impact the success of your fitness program. If the intensity at which you exercise is too low, you won't burn as much fat as you could. If it's too high, you risk injury. The American College of Sports Medicine recommends that most people exercise at an intensity level that ranges between 55 and 90 percent of their maximum heart rate. For a more detailed explanation, see "More on Intensity," below.

TIME (DURATION): *Time* refers to how *long* you work out. In general, you must raise your heart rate for at least 20 minutes to give your cardiovascular system an adequate workout. I recommend 30 to 40 minutes of cardio, which includes warmup and cooldown periods. Have a hard time finding the time to exercise? Good news: Research suggests that even short bursts of physical activity accumulated throughout the day can be as beneficial as longer exercise sessions. So if you can't spend a full 30 minutes on the treadmill or bike, jump on three times a day for 10 minutes. *Beginners:* Start with 10 to 15 minutes at a time, including your warmup and cooldown, and increase this duration by 2 minutes per week until you have exceeded 20 minutes.

MORE ON INTENSITY

To boost your weight loss as well as your fitness level, you must perform cardio within your *target heart rate (THR)* zone. Your THR is 55 to 90 percent of your *maximum heart rate (MHR)*. Based on your age, MHR is the upper limit of what your cardiovascular system can handle during physical activity, and it's different for everyone.

To check your heart rate during exercise, briefly stop your activity and take your pulse at the wrist. Place the tips of your index and middle fingers (not your thumb) over the artery in your wrist and press lightly. Take a full 60-second count of the heartbeats, or take it for 30 seconds and multiply by 2. Start the count on a beat, which is counted as "zero."

Below, you'll learn how to find your target heart rate and be given guidelines on how intensely to work out based on your fitness level.

THE LOW-INTENSITY ZONE (NOVICE): Keep your THR between 50 and 60 percent of your maximum heart rate. This is the easiest and most comfortable level of intensity for exercise and it's great for warmups and cooldowns. While you'll burn the fewest calories in this zone, you still can reap cardiorespiratory benefits and reduce your body fat, blood pressure, and cholesterol.

To estimate whether you are working in the low-intensity range, subtract your age from 220 to arrive at your MHR. For example, if you're 40 years old, your estimated MHR is 220–40 years = 180 beats per minute (bpm). The 50 and 60 percent levels would be:

- ♣ 50 percent level: $180 \times 0.50 = 90$ bpm
- ♣ 60 percent level: $180 \times 0.60 = 108$ bpm

Low-intensity physical activity would keep your heart rate between 90 and 108 bpm.

THE MODERATE-INTENSITY ZONE (SKILLED AND MASTER): Keep your THR between 65 and 70 percent of your MHR. If you've been working out for at least 6 months and want to burn fat, stick to this zone: Roughly 85 percent of the calories burned in the moderate-intensity zone are from fat. You'll burn more calories than you would in the low-intensity zone. To use our example above, a 40-year-old's THR would be:

- ♣ 65 percent level: $180 \times 0.65 = 117$ bpm
- ♣ 70 percent level: $180 \times 0.70 = 126$ bpm

THE HIGH-INTENSITY ZONE (SKILLED AND MASTER): Keep your THR between 75 and 85 percent of your MHR. This zone improves your cardiovascular and respiratory systems and actually increases the size and strength of your heart. As your endurance improves, you can exercise for longer. The more exercise you can do, the more calories you'll burn and the more body fat you'll lose. It's true that in this zone you burn fewer calories from fat, *but* you burn more total calories than in the other zones. This high-intensity zone is also best for interval training.

Again, if you're 40 years old, calculate your THR this way:

- ❖ 75 percent level: $180 \times 0.75 = 135$ bpm

- ❖ 85 percent level: $180 \times 0.85 = 153$ bpm

A high-intensity workout requires that your THR remain between 135 and 153 bpm during physical activity.

If you're just starting my program, keep your THR at the lower end of your zone and gradually work up to a higher intensity level. Also, talk to your doctor before you begin this or any exercise program. If you have heart disease, high blood pressure, or another chronic health condition, he or she may recommend a lower THR zone. But don't worry—even at the lower limits, you'll still reap the benefits of regular cardio-vascular exercise.

MONITORING YOUR HEART RATE

Whatever your fitness level, you must exercise at the right intensity to get results. There are two ways to determine whether you're reaching—and maintaining—the correct level of intensity during your workout.

The first way is with a heart-rate monitor, available at sporting-goods stores and department stores. It's a simple device: A wireless strap that goes around your chest continuously measures your heart rate, which is displayed on a wristwatch-like device. When you increase or reduce your effort, it reflects the resulting change in your heart rate.

The second, low-tech way is to use the Talk Test, which monitors your ability to talk during your workout. If you are working at *low* intensity, you should be able to sing. If you are working at a *moderate* level of intensity, you should be able to comfortably carry on a conversation. If you are too out of breath to speak, you are engaged in *high-intensity* activity.

I recommend that you team the Talk Test with your rate of perceived exertion (RPE). While a heart-rate monitor can be helpful in establishing a target zone, I prefer to tune in to my body's response to various levels of cardio intensity rather than depend solely on the number on a heart-rate monitor. The body always knows best—it will tell you how much effort it can handle.

The standard measure of RPE, the Borg Rate of Perceived Exertion Scale, measures your perception of how intensely you are exercising. I believe simpler is better, so I have devised a condensed version of the scale. For all interval sessions, judge your exertion on this scale of 1 to 9, with 1 being snoozing and 9 being on the verge of collapse. *Note: Do not exceed a level of 8 (preferably 7) in your cardio sessions.*

LEVEL 1: NO INTENSITY. You could be napping.

LEVEL 2: VERY LIGHT INTENSITY. You could maintain this pace all day and easily talk your head off on a cell phone.

LEVEL 3: MODERATELY LIGHT INTENSITY. You can easily carry on a conversation.

LEVEL 4: MODERATE INTENSITY. You're breathing more heavily. Talking requires some effort.

LEVEL 5: SOMEWHAT HARD INTENSITY. You're breathing heavily and sweating more. Talking requires more effort.

LEVEL 6: HARD INTENSITY. Conversation is challenging.

LEVEL 7: VERY HARD INTENSITY. You are breathing heavily, sweating a lot, and grunting your words. You can keep this pace up for 60 seconds or less.

LEVEL 8: EXTREMELY HARD INTENSITY. Talking isn't an option. You're working too hard.

LEVEL 9: MAXIMUM INTENSITY. You are huffing, puffing, and gasping for breath. Never strive for, or reach, this level of effort during a cardio session.

HIGH AND LOW, FAST AND SLOW

Research shows that vigorous bursts of cardio followed by easier ones burn more calories in less time than exercising at a steady intensity. This technique, called *interval training*, involves the use of set "intervals"—often measured in time—that dictate the intensity of training. In a nutshell, you exercise at high intensity for a specific distance or time, briefly lower the intensity so you can recover, then return to the high-intensity interval. This method is repeated numerous times in one cardio session.

PHYSICAL ACTIVITIES DEFINED BY LEVEL OF INTENSITY*

MODERATE ACTIVITY

Walking, moderate or brisk pace
(3–4½ mph), level surface

Hiking

Roller-skating or in-line skating,
leisurely pace

Bicycling, 5–9 mph, level terrain
or a few hills

Stationary bicycling, moderate effort

Aerobic dancing, low impact

Aquatic aerobics

Calisthenics, light

Yoga

Gymnastics

Jumping on a trampoline

Stairclimber machine,
light or moderate pace

Rowing machine, moderate effort

Weight training (free weights,
Nautilus- or Universal-type weights)

Dancing (ballet, ballroom,
line, square, folk, modern)

Tennis (doubles)

Golf, wheeling or carrying clubs

Frisbee

Badminton

Downhill skiing, light effort

Ice-skating, leisurely pace

Swimming, recreational

VIGOROUS ACTIVITY

Racewalking or aerobic walking,
5 mph or faster

Jogging or running

Backpacking

Mountain climbing or rock climbing

Roller-skating or in-line skating, brisk pace

Bicycling, 10 mph or greater
or on steep terrain

Stationary bicycling, vigorous effort

Aerobic dancing, high impact

Step aerobics

Aquatic jogging

Calisthenics, vigorous effort

Martial arts

Jumping rope

Stairclimber machine, fast pace

Rowing machine, vigorous effort

Circuit weight training

Dancing, energetic
(ballroom, line, square, folk)

Tennis (singles), racquetball, squash

Downhill skiing, vigorous effort

Ice-skating, fast pace

Cross-country skiing

Sledding or tobogganing

Swimming, steady paced laps

Aquatic polo or basketball

*Adapted from guidelines developed by the Centers for
Disease Control and the American College of Sports Medicine.*

Interval training adds variety to a workout, increases the number of calories you burn, and makes your cardio fly by—constantly cranking up and slowing down the intensity takes your mind off of how long you've been working out. Intervals also challenge your whole body because the varying intensities or movements require your body to use different muscles. This means you get a better overall workout.

In my program, you can choose interval training or maintain an even intensity level during the bulk of your workout (a method called *long, steady distance training*). If you opt for intervals, your cardio sessions will last 30 minutes. If you choose long, steady distance training, you will work out for 40 minutes. Several rules apply, however.

❧ If you're a Novice, perform intervals no more than 3 days per week on nonconsecutive days.

❧ If you are starting at the Skilled or Master level and choose to perform cardio only 3 days per week, choose interval style and perform it on nonconsecutive days.

❧ If you are at Skilled or Master level and choose to perform cardio 5 days per week, you should still stick to 3 days of intervals, along with 2 days of long, steady cardio.

❧ Regardless of your fitness level, practice intervals in moderation, because too much high-intensity exercise can lead to injury.

The following guidelines factor in your current level of fitness.

NOVICE (YOU ARE NEW TO EXERCISE): Alternate 1-minute high-intensity intervals with 3-minute recovery intervals.

SKILLED OR MASTER (YOU HAVE PERFORMED CARDIO FOR AT LEAST 6 MONTHS): Alternate high-intensity intervals of 90 to 120 seconds with 2-minute recovery intervals. Or push even harder by alternating 30-second high-intensity intervals with recovery intervals of 90 seconds.

This is how my scale might work for a typical 30-minute interval cardio session.

MINUTES 1 TO 5: Warm up with one of my suggested warmups, or walk at a pace of 3 or 4 on my modified RPE scale (see page 11).

MINUTES 6 TO 26: Maintain a steady pace within the 4 to 6 range. *Optional:* Alternate higher-intensity (6 or 7 RPE) 1-minute intervals with lower-intensity (4 or 5 RPE) 2-minute recovery intervals. For the high-intensity intervals, start at the lower range of intensity (6, for example) early in your workout, gradually build to a higher range of intensity (7) toward the middle of your session, then drop back down again near the end of your workout. On the recovery intervals, choose the lower range (4, for example) if the high-intensity interval wore you out or the higher range (5) if you still feel energetic.

MINUTES 27 TO 30: To cool down, perform one of my suggested cooldowns, or walk at a pace of 3 or 4 on my modified RPE scale.

If you can do only 20 minutes of cardio, perform a 5-minute warmup followed by steady intensity within the 4 to 6 range for minutes 6 through 17. *Optional:* Alternate four higher-intensity (6 or 7 RPE) intervals with four lower-intensity (4 or 5 RPE) recovery intervals, then perform a 3-minute cooldown.

WALK THIS WAY

Walking is the most popular form of cardio—it's simple, inexpensive, and fun. To get the most from your walk, follow these guidelines. (If you have a chronic health condition such as heart disease or diabetes, check with your doctor before taking your first step.)

WALK BRISKLY for 3 to 5 minutes at a pace that is at a 3 or 4 RPE.

AFTER YOUR WARMUP, PERFORM TOE RAISES AND ANKLE ROLLS. *Toe raises:* Stand in place. With one foot at a time, raise your toes, flexing your foot and keeping your heel on the ground. Lower your toes and repeat. Perform 8 to 12 repetitions per foot; try to increase the range of motion with each repetition. *Ankle rolls:* Sit or stand, holding the back of a bench or sturdy chair for balance, if you like. Lift one foot off the ground. Roll it clockwise at the ankle for 8 to 12 repetitions, then counterclockwise for 8 to 12 repetitions. Switch feet.

STRIKE THE GROUND WITH YOUR HEEL FIRST. Lift your toes without locking your knees and roll through your arches, pushing off from the ball of your foot to propel your body forward. Avoid hitting the ground with a slap.

BEND YOUR ELBOWS AT A 90-DEGREE ANGLE. Keep them close to your sides and swing your arms back and forth in opposition to your leg motion. The correct swinging technique is to drive your elbow back and behind you, then bring it back up to your rib cage.

AS YOU WALK, STAND ERECT, KEEP YOUR HEAD UP, AND FOCUS ON A POINT 10 TO 20 FEET AHEAD. Also, contract your abdominal muscles and keep your shoulders down and away from your ears.

TO WALK FASTER, TAKE SHORTER, QUICKER STEPS. Push off with your toes, land on your heel, and roll through the step.

TO BURN MORE CALORIES, alternate between a brisk pace and 30-second intervals at an even more intense pace.

TREAT YOURSELF TO GOOD WALKING SHOES. They are designed to help propel you through the heel-toe motion of the proper walking technique and can help prevent walking-related injuries such as knee problems. Buy them from an experienced salesperson at a specialty running-shoe store.

PURCHASE A PEDOMETER. This inexpensive little gadget clips onto your belt or waistband and tracks the number of steps you take during the day—a fun, easy, and inexpensive form of motivation.

IF YOU WALK OUTSIDE, dress in weather-appropriate layers. The layer closest to your skin should be made of a fabric such as polypropylene that will wick sweat away from your skin. (Cotton holds sweat next to the skin.) The next layer should insulate—a shirt or hoodie that can easily be removed when you warm up, for example. For your outer layer, don a light jacket—windproof for cooler weather, waterproof or water-resistant for wet weather.

IF YOU WALK AT NIGHT, invest in a mesh reflective safety vest, available at biking or running shops.

SPICE UP YOUR TREADMILL WORKOUT

Like many folks, I do my cardio on a treadmill. But because the pounding of running makes my back hurt and tightens my hips, I created this 30-minute treadmill routine. Now, I'm passing it on to you. Some of the moves can be tricky at first, but that's a good thing, especially if your current treadmill workout feels a bit stale. As you learn this routine, feel free to walk, jog, or run instead of doing any of the moves.

MINUTES 1 TO 5: WARMUP WITH UPPER BODY MOVES

❖ **WARMUP.** Holding the rails or handles of your treadmill with both hands, round your upper back for a few steps. Straighten up, then lift your chest toward the ceiling for a few steps. Repeat 3 to 5 times.

❖ **SINGLE-ARM REACHES.** Keeping one hand on the rail or bar, extend your other arm straight over your head as you walk. Lower it, then repeat with your other arm. Try to reach higher with each rep. Do 10 to 20 alternating reaches.

❖ **BEND DOWN LOW.** Walk briskly for 10 to 20 steps. Then bend your knees slightly and walk in this fashion at the same pace for 10 to 20 steps, keeping your upper body upright. Alternate between brisk walking and bent-knee walking. Repeat 3 to 5 times.

MINUTES 6 TO 25: SPEED UP AND CHANGE UP

❖ **MINUTES 6 TO 8.** Fitness walk: Increase your pace to a level 4 or 5 RPE (see page 11 for the RPE scale). Walk briskly.

❖ **MINUTES 9 TO 10.** Step-step-sashay: Step forward with your right foot, then your left foot. Then sashay: Step forward again with your right foot and hop to bring your left foot to meet your right, landing first on your left foot and then your right foot. Immediately step forward with your left foot and hop to bring your right foot to meet your left, landing first on your right foot, then your left foot. Continue to alternate sashays after each two regular steps forward. Before you try sashays on the treadmill, be sure you can do them on the floor or other nonmoving surface!

❖ **MINUTES 11 TO 14.** Step-togethers: Think of this move as walking sideways in a straight line. Raise the incline to 3.0 (Novice)–6.0 (Master). *Novice:* Reduce the treadmill's speed to 1.8–2.0 mph. *Skilled:* Reduce the treadmill's speed to 2.0–2.5 mph. *Master:* Set the speed as you see fit. Hold the rail or bar with your left hand and turn your body to the right, so that your left shoulder is closest to the bar and your body is a quarter turn to the right. Leading with your left foot, step to the side and then bring your right foot to meet your left. Do step-togethers on one side for minutes 11 and 12, walk forward briskly for a few seconds, then switch to the other side for the remainder of minutes 13 and 14. Advanced exercisers can try hopping together instead of stepping together.

✤ **MINUTES 15 TO 18.** Keep the treadmill set at a 3.0–6.0 incline. Side-squat walking: Facing a quarter turn to the right on the treadmill, place your hands on your thighs, bend your knees, and lower yourself into a step-together. Hold a half-squat position as you walk sideways with your left foot leading. Do side-squat walking leading with the left foot for minutes 15 and 16, walk forward briskly for a few seconds, then switch to the other side for the remainder of minutes 17 and 18.

✤ **MINUTES 19 TO 21.** Depending on your fitness level, keep the incline up or reduce it. Walk briskly as you hold your arms straight over your head. For less of a challenge, place your hands behind your head. This less-difficult variation still forces your core to work harder and makes a nice little abs workout.

✤ **MINUTES 22 TO 24.** Incline walking: In accordance with your fitness level, walk, jog, or run on an incline of 3, 4, or 5 to work your glutes and hamstrings.

✤ **MINUTE 25.** *Novice:* Lower the incline and perform one last blast of fitness walking. *Skilled* and *Master:* Keep an incline, but reduce the treadmill's speed (to 1.8–2.5 mph for Novice and Skilled levels and up to 3.0 mph for Master). Holding the bars or rails, *carefully* turn 180 degrees so that your back is to the rail or bar and you are walking "backward." Hold on to the rail or bars as you walk backward—you'll feel a burn in the front of your thighs. Carefully turn until you're facing forward.

MINUTES 26 TO 30: COOLDOWN

✤ **REPEAT THE WARMUP.** Reduce the treadmill's incline. Slow your pace even more until you are walking very slowly. Shake one leg, step, step, shake the other leg, step, step. Repeat until you've shaken each leg 10 to 20 times.

✤ **TAKE TWO DEEP BREATHS.** Extend both arms over your head on the inhalation and lower them on the exhalation.

❖

STRETCH YOURSELF:
FLEXIBILITY TRAINING FOR TOTAL BODY FITNESS

Toned muscles and a strong heart are only part of the fitness equation. If you're not flexible, you're not truly fit. That's why, with my program, you limber up as you slim down.

Flexibility training boosts your energy level, maintains your youthful posture, prevents injuries, and de-stresses your mind and body. But if you haven't heard of it, you're not alone. Unfortunately, some fitness programs minimize its importance, emphasizing fat loss and muscle gain over joint mobility.

In our "chair-bound" society, however, maintaining flexibility is crucial, and it becomes even more important as we age. Maintaining your flexibility will protect your ability to perform activities you may take for granted today, such as dressing and reaching the top shelf of your kitchen cabinets. Flexibility is independence. To be flexible is to be open, pliable, durable, youthful, balanced, *empowered*. Flexibility is the gateway to health, happiness, and well-being.

Think I'm overstating things? No way. If your goal is total fitness, flexibility training is just as important as strength training, cardiovascular exercise, balance practice, and core work. Leaving flexibility training out of your fitness program is like eliminating healthy carbohydrates from your diet. Imbalances in your body would develop and hinder your results or, worse, cause injury.

But what *is* flexibility, anyway? Quite simply, it's the ability to move your joints and muscles through their full range of motion (ROM). A joint is the point of connection between two bones. A joint's ROM, or flexibility, depends on the stretchiness of the surrounding muscles and tendons. Thus, it is critical to stretch the muscles that surround a joint to increase the ROM your joint can move through.

The average person can expect to lose 70 percent of her flexibility between the ages of 20 and 70. While a lack of flexibility may not be life threatening, it can be debilitating. With decreased flexibility, joint stiffness sets in and muscles lose their pliability—an uncomfortable, limiting, and potentially painful way to live.

The good news? There's much you can do to stay limber and flexible well into old age. That's why flexibility training is an essential and required component of my 4-week intensive program. The most important benefit of any flexibility program is prevention of injury. But there are plenty of other benefits, too. Consistent flexibility training, properly performed, can:

❖ even out the body's muscular strengths and weaknesses

❖ give the body a more symmetrical appearance

❖ alleviate muscle soreness and promote faster recovery from workouts

❖ promote relaxation

❖ release emotional stress manifested deep within the tissues

❖ improve posture by balancing muscle groups that might be overused during exercise

THERE'S MORE THAN ONE WAY TO STRETCH

Do you think stretching is just for marathon runners or yoga aficionados? Think again. There are several types of stretching techniques. In this book, I ask you to perform two kinds of stretches. The first is called *static*; the second, *moving flexibility*.

In static stretching, you hold a stretch without moving for 10 for 30 seconds. Static stretching is quite relaxing—it's a great way to end a workout, especially if you've pushed yourself hard. With moving flexibility stretches, you stretch a muscle, or a group of muscles, by contracting an opposing muscle group or groups.

I believe that both styles of stretching are important. Static stretching can be easier—you don't have to think about anything beyond the muscle you're stretching. Moving flexibility stretching requires you to focus on alignment, form, posture, and so forth. You'll work harder, but one session of moving flexibility stretching, properly performed, is at least twice as effective as one session of static stretching.

Because moving flexibility stretches are as much about strength as they are about flexibility, however, at the end of a tough workout you may want to perform the less challenging static stretches. That said, if you want to do moving flexibility stretches at the end of an intense workout, go for it! The bottom line: Listen to your body and choose the appropriate type of stretch.

THE STRETCHES

You will stretch at the beginning and end of your workout, and between sets of each move.

BEFORE YOUR WORKOUT: Start with one of my 3-minute total body warmups (see page 14 or 16).

DURING YOUR WORKOUT: Between each set, perform the static and moving flexibility stretches recommended with each move. Moving flexibility exercises stimulate your blood's circulation, which means that your muscles will receive more blood and nutrients as they work and will recover more quickly for the next set. The static stretches help to increase muscle flexibility, promote relaxation, and alleviate post-workout soreness.

AFTER YOUR WORKOUT: Perform my cooldown routine (see page 17).

STATIC STRETCHES	MOVING FLEXIBILITY STRETCHES
Seated Forward Bend	Chair Pose to Standing Forward Bend
Reaching Butterfly	Split Leg
Kneeling Lunge (static version)	Kneeling Lunge (moving flexibility version)
Single-Arm Reach Across (static version)	Lying Split Leg
Modified Hurdler	Single-Arm Reach Across (moving flexibility version)
Standing Quadriceps	Bent-Arm Overhead
One-Arm Round Front	Single-Arm Reach Back
Child's Pose with Reach Across (static version)	Walking Quadriceps
Spinal Twist	Open Arm
Cobra Pose	Child's Pose with Reach Across (moving flexibility version)
	Lunge with One-Arm Reach
	Child's Pose to Upward-Facing Dog

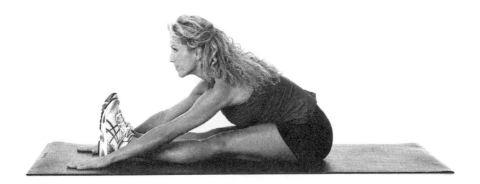

SEATED FORWARD BEND

This move stretches the hamstrings and calves.

Sit tall on your sit bones on the floor with your shoulders and hips squared and aligned. Placing your arms at your sides with your palms on the floor, extend your legs straight in front of you. Contract your abdominal muscles. Slowly walk your hands alongside your legs as far toward your toes as you can. The stretch should feel good, not hurt. Inhale and exhale deeply through your nose, trying to go deeper into the stretch with each exhalation. Hold the stretch for 10 to 30 seconds.

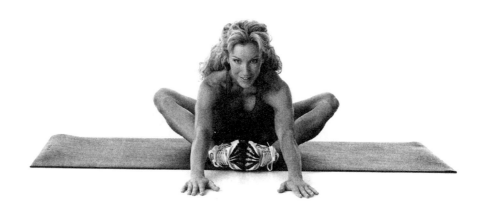

REACHING BUTTERFLY

This move stretches your lower back, inner thighs, and glutes.

Sit tall on your sit bones on the floor and square your hips and shoulders. Drop your knees to your sides so that the soles of your feet face each other. If you are flexible enough, touch your soles together, or keep them 5 to 10 inches apart. Extend your arms in front of you and as far past your legs as you can. Experiment with the spacing of your feet—closer together, farther apart—to find the position that delivers the maximum stretch in your lower back. Hold for 10 to 30 seconds, breathing deeply.

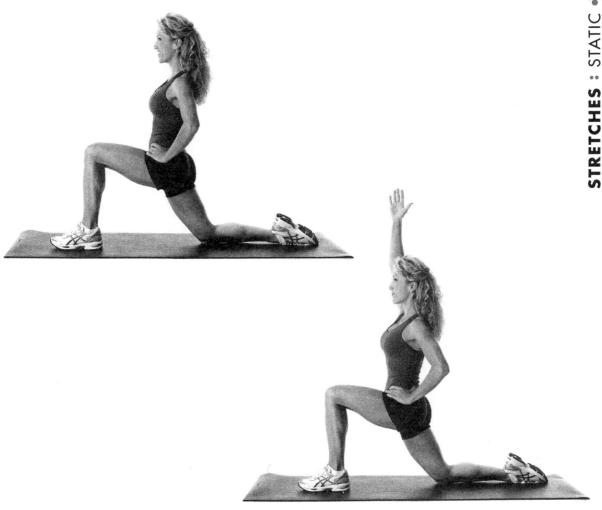

KNEELING LUNGE

This move stretches the quadriceps, hip flexors, hamstrings, and glutes.

Kneel with one side of your body next to a wall or sturdy chair. (Kneel on a towel, if you like.) Square your hips and shoulders. Raise your left leg and bring it forward, placing your left foot 2 feet in front of your right knee. Contract your right glutes (the muscles of the buttocks) and press your right hip forward. For added stretch, extend your right arm over your head. Hold for 10 to 30 seconds (remember to breathe!). Switch to the opposite leg and repeat.

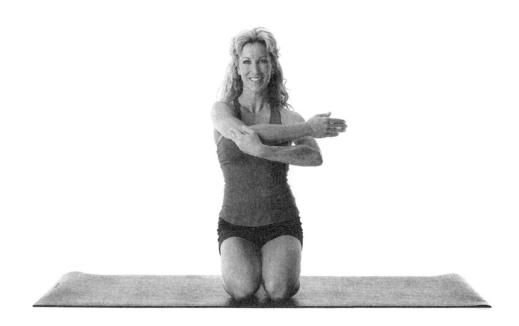

SINGLE-ARM REACH ACROSS
This move stretches the deltoids (shoulders).

Stand or sit or kneel and lift your right arm to shoulder height in front of you. Bring your arm as far across your chest as you can. Place your left palm on your right elbow to pull your right arm closer to your chest. Hold for 10 to 30 seconds, breathing deeply, then switch sides and repeat.

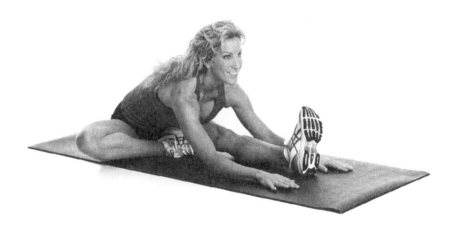

MODIFIED HURDLER

This move stretches the hamstrings, glutes, and lower back.

Sit tall on your sit bones with your left leg extended in front of you. Bend your right knee and bring the sole of your right foot to your left inner thigh. Reach with both hands for your left foot and bend your torso toward your left leg. If you can reach your left foot, grasp the sole and gently extend your torso toward it. Hold for 10 to 30 seconds, breathing deeply throughout, then switch sides and repeat.

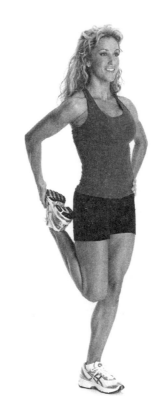

STANDING QUADRICEPS

This move stretches the quadriceps and hip flexors and improves balance.
Novices: If you find yourself losing your balance, hold on to the back of a
chair or a wall.

Stand with your feet hip-width apart; contract your abdominal muscles. Raise your right
foot off the floor and bend your leg to the rear, bringing your heel as close as you can to
your glutes. Grasp your right foot with your right hand and pull your heel even closer.
Hold for 10 to 30 seconds, then switch sides and repeat.

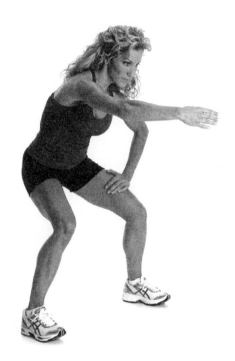

ONE-ARM ROUND FRONT

This move stretches the entire back and strengthens the abdominal muscles.

Stand with your feet wider than shoulder-width apart, knees bent, and abdominals contracted. Place your left hand on your left thigh. Raise your right arm to the front and left, rounding it as if you were holding a beach ball. Round your back like a cat; feel the stretch between your shoulder blades and all the way down your spine. Breathe deeply and hold the stretch for 10 to 30 seconds. Switch arms and repeat.

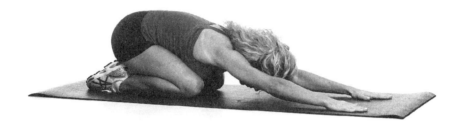

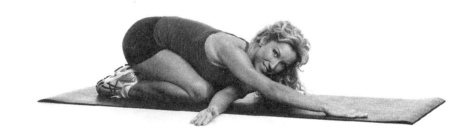

CHILD'S POSE
WITH **REACH ACROSS**

*This stretch stretches the back and shoulders
and rests the body after an intense move.*

Kneel on the floor. Extend both arms toward the floor and lower yourself so that your
upper legs are folded over your lower legs, your forehead rests comfortably on or near the
floor, and your arms on the floor extend beyond your head. You are in Child's Pose. Hold
for 10 to 30 seconds, breathing deeply. Then, bend your left elbow and reach with your
left arm, palm up, beneath and across your body to your right side. Depending on your
flexibility level, you may need to slightly raise your torso off the floor. You should feel a
stretch in your left shoulder. Hold, breathing deeply, for 10 to 30 seconds. Switch arms
and hold for 10 to 30 seconds.

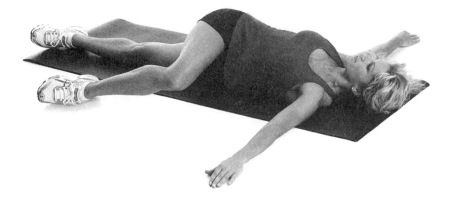

SPINAL TWIST

This stretch stretches the entire back and relieves tension in the lower back.

Lie on your back with your your legs straight out on the floor. Extend your arms straight out to the sides at shoulder height. Bend your right knee and lift your right leg off the floor until your right calf is parallel to the floor with your right knee lined up over your right hip. Next, lower your right knee to the left until it touches the floor, keeping your torso facing the ceiling. Hold, breathing deeply, for 10 to 30 seconds. Return to the starting position and repeat with your left leg, lowering your knee to the right. Hold for 10 to 30 seconds.

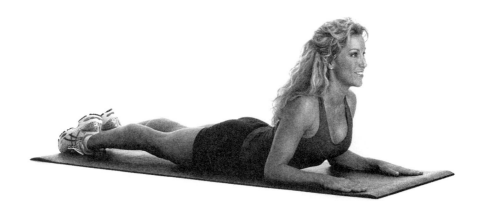

COBRA POSE

This move stretches the chest, shoulders, neck, and abs.
It also strengthens the back (the erector spinae muscles).

Lie on your stomach with your body in a long, straight line. Place your hands, palms down, on the floor by your shoulders. Using your back muscles and lightly assisting with your palms, lift your head, shoulders, and chest off the floor. Lift as high as you can without compressing your spine. As you lift, picture your head reaching for the ceiling. Feel the stretch in your neck and abdominals. Hold for 5 to 10 seconds, breathing deeply, then lower your torso to the floor.

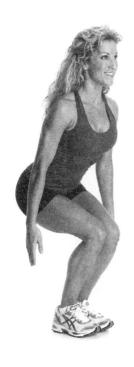
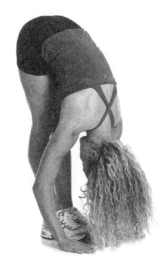

CHAIR POSE TO STANDING FORWARD BEND

This stretch stretches the hamstrings and glutes, opens the spine, relaxes the back, strengthens the quadriceps and lower back muscles, and improves balance.

Stand with your feet together, arms at your sides. Contract your abdominal muscles, draw your navel toward your spine, and align your hips and shoulders. Bend your knees and lower yourself into a squat, as if you are going to sit in a chair. (This is the Chair Pose.) Hold for 3 to 5 seconds, then, bending forward at the waist, lower your torso toward your thighs as you straighten your legs and stand. (This is the Standing Forward Bend.) From this position, try to place your palms flat on the floor. If you can't fully straighten your legs, softly bend your knees. Keeping your quadriceps contracted, lift your tailbone toward the ceiling. Hold for 3 to 5 seconds, then bend your knees and return to the Chair Pose. Hold for 3 to 5 seconds, then repeat the forward bend. Alternate poses, moving slowly from one to the other, until you have performed each one 3 to 5 times. Breathe deeply through your nose and try to go deeper into the Standing Forward Bend with each repetition.

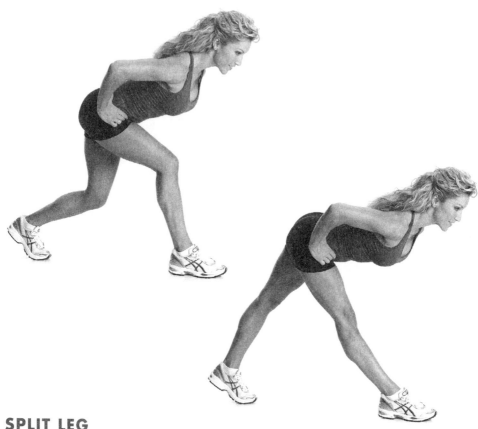

SPLIT LEG

This stretch stretches the hamstrings and glutes and tones the quadriceps, hip flexors, and abdominal muscles.

Stand with your feet hip-width apart. Take a giant step backward with your left foot, distributing your weight equally between both feet and bending both knees 1 to 3 inches. Put your hands on your hips. Lower your torso toward your right leg, straightening your knees and lifting your tailbone toward the ceiling. (If you can't straighten your knees, keep them slightly bent.) Continue to contract your quadriceps and abdominals to help you maintain your balance. You should feel a stretch in your hamstrings. Next, keeping your torso lowered, bend both knees 1 to 3 inches. Then straighten both legs again, trying to lift your tailbone higher toward the ceiling. Perform 5 slow reps and switch legs. If you need help balancing, hold on to the back of a sturdy chair.

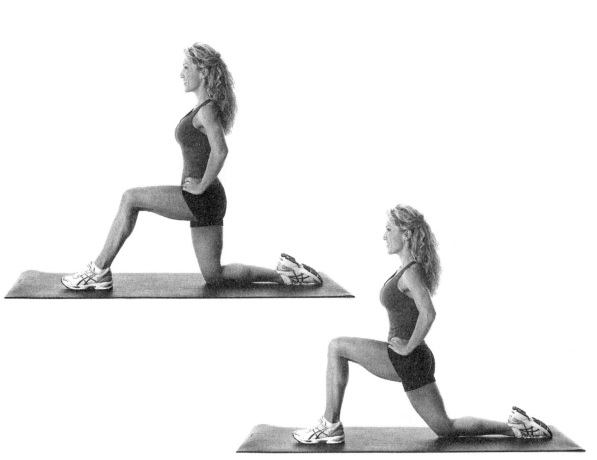

KNEELING LUNGE

This stretch stretches the quadriceps, hip flexors, hamstrings, and glutes.

Perform 5 slow repetitions of the Kneeling Lunge (page 25), exhaling as you press forward with your left hip and inhaling as you release. Then switch sides and perform 5 repetitions on the other side.

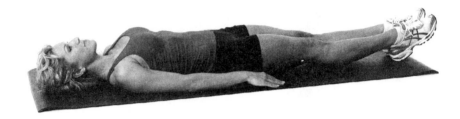

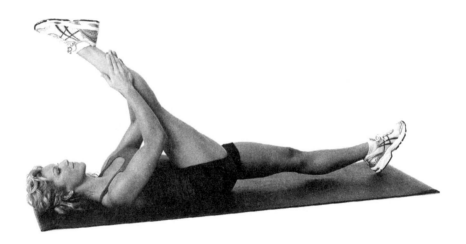

LYING SPLIT LEG

This stretch stretches the hamstrings and glutes,
strengthens the quadriceps, and alleviates lower back pain.

Lie on your back. Keeping your left leg straight, contract and use your quadriceps to lift your right leg as high as you can toward your chest. When you cannot get your leg any closer to your chest, grasp your right calf and gently pull your leg 2 to 3 inches closer, exhaling as you do so. Lower your leg and repeat. Try to lift your leg a bit further each time, as well as pull it a bit closer to your chest. Perform 5 to 10 repetitions, exhaling as you lift and pull and inhaling as you lower your leg. Switch sides and repeat.

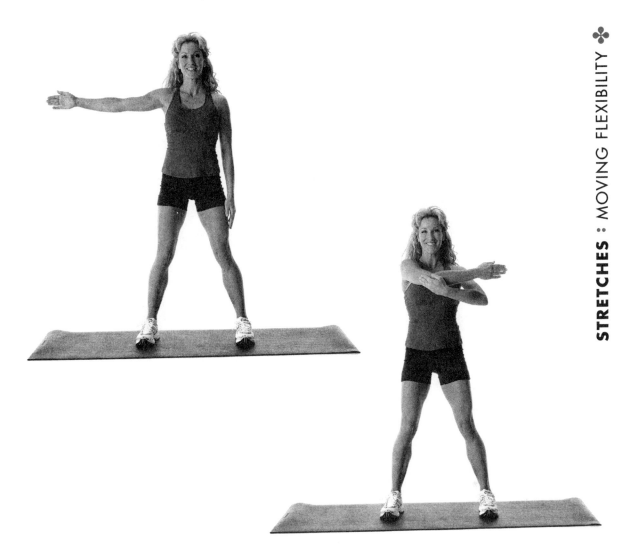

SINGLE-ARM REACH ACROSS

This stretch stretches the deltoids (shoulders).

Stand or sit and extend your right arm out to the side at shoulder height. Using your chest muscles, bring your arm as far across your chest as you can, exhaling as you do so. Then assist the stretch by pulling your right arm closer to your chest with your left hand, continuing to exhale. Inhale as you return your arm to the starting position. Repeat for a total of 8 to 12 reps, then switch sides and repeat.

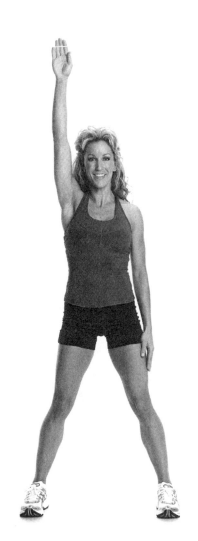
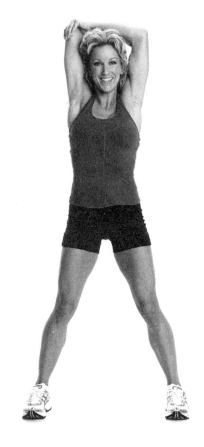

BENT-ARM OVERHEAD

This stretch stretches the triceps, latissimus dorsi, and rear deltoids.

Stand or sit tall. Inhale, raise your right arm alongside your ear, and bend your elbow, allowing your forearm to drop behind your head. Using your left hand, grasp your right elbow and gently pull your arm to the left behind your head, exhaling as you do so. Hold for 2 to 3 seconds, then lower your right arm back to the starting position. Repeat 5 to 10 times, trying for a deeper stretch with each repetition. Switch sides and complete 5 to 10 reps on the other side.

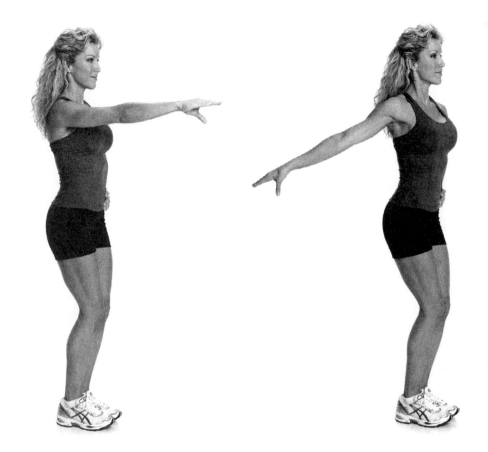

SINGLE-ARM REACH BACK

This stretch stretches the biceps, shoulders, and chest muscles
and strengthens the rear deltoid and upper back muscles.

Stand or sit on the floor. Extend your right arm in front of you at shoulder height, palm down. Shape your hand like the wide-open jaws of a crocodile: index to pinkie fingers together, thumb separate. Sweep your arm out to the side and then behind your body, extending through your fingertips as you maintain the crocodile-jaw hand position (it correctly aligns the biceps for stretching). Then, return your arm to the starting position and repeat. Exhale as you reach back; inhale as you return to the starting position. Perform 5 to 10 reps per arm.

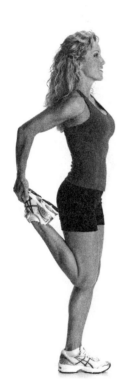 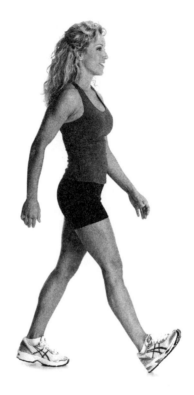 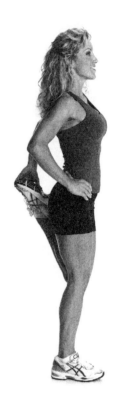

WALKING QUADRICEPS

This stretch stretches the quadriceps and hip flexors.

Stand with your feet hip-width apart; contract your abdominal muscles. Step forward with your left foot and bend and raise your right knee to the rear, using your hamstring to bring your right heel as close to your glutes as you can. Then, assist the stretch: Grasp your right foot with your right hand and pull your heel even closer. Then, lower your right foot and immediately step forward on it to allow you to lift your left foot to perform the stretch. Perform 1 set of 10 to 20 alternating stretches. Inhale as you step forward; exhale as you pull on your foot.

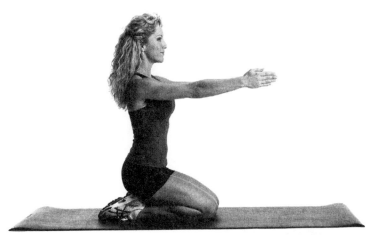

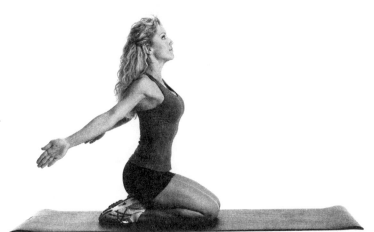

OPEN ARM

This stretch stretches the shoulders and chest and tones and stretches the upper back.

Stand or kneel, resting your butt on the backs of your heels. Lift your arms to shoulder height in front of you, arms straight and palms facing each other. Draw your shoulders back and down and sweep your arms to the side and as far behind you as you can, exhaling as you do so. (It's fine if your arms drop a bit below shoulder height as you stretch.) Then, use your chest and shoulder muscles to bring your arms forward to the starting position, touching your hands together. Repeat for a total of 8 to 12 repetitions.

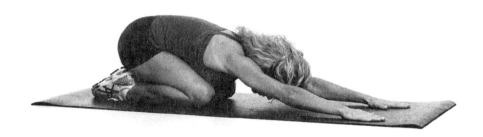

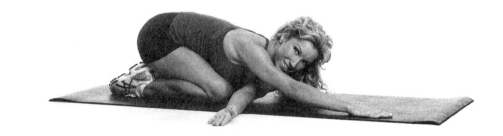

CHILD'S POSE WITH REACH ACROSS

This stretch stretches the back and shoulders and strengthens the chest and abs.

Begin in Child's Pose (page 30). Bend your left elbow and reach with your left arm, palm up, beneath your torso and across your body to your right side; straighten your arm, palm still facing toward the ceiling. You should feel a stretch in your left shoulder. Hold for 2 seconds. Return your left arm to the starting position and switch arms, moving your right arm beneath and across your body. Hold for 2 seconds. Continue alternating arms for 3 to 5 repetitions per side. Breathe deeply and move slowly.

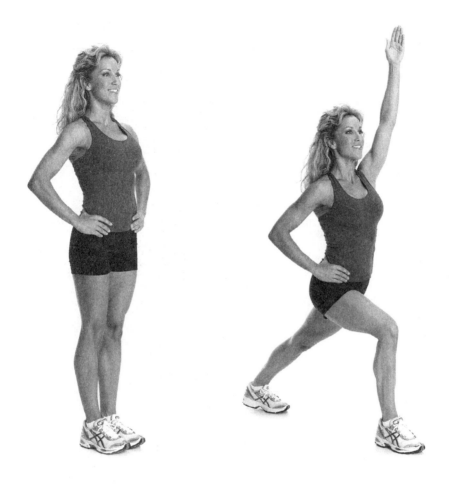

LUNGE WITH ONE-ARM REACH

This move stretches the hip flexors and abdominals and strengthens the back, glutes, and hamstrings.

Stand with your feet together and your hands on your hips. Contract your abdominals and align your hips and shoulders. Inhale, then exhale as you take a big step backward with your left foot. Keep your left leg straight but bend your right (front) knee. Raise your left arm as high as you can and press your left hip downward so that you really lengthen your torso. Return to the starting position and switch sides. Perform 10 to 20 alternating reps in a slow, controlled manner, reaching and extending further with each rep.

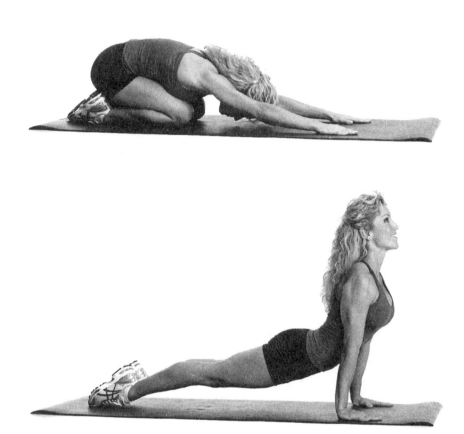

CHILD'S POSE TO UPWARD-FACING DOG

*This move stretches the abdominals, hip flexors,
chest, shoulders, and neck and relaxes the body.*

Assume the Child's Pose (see page 30); hold for 3 seconds, inhaling deeply. Pull yourself forward and unfold your body, continuing to contract your abdominals as you straighten your legs and lift your torso toward the ceiling, supporting yourself on your hands, positioned directly below your shoulders. Hold the Upward-Facing Dog position for 3 seconds, exhaling deeply. Push backward and return to the Child's Pose. Move slowly from pose to pose 5 to 10 times, exhaling as you move into the Upward-Facing Dog and inhaling as you return to the Child's Pose.

FLEXIBILITY FACTORS

AGE. As we age, our muscles tend to shorten due to a lack of physical activity and a loss of elasticity in the connective tissues around the muscles. The result is some loss of flexibility.

GENDER. Throughout their lives, women tend to be more flexible than men of a similar age, generally due to anatomical variations in joints.

EXERCISE. Participation in regular exercise involving a full range of motion tends to increase flexibility; a sedentary lifestyle tends to reduce it.

TYPE OF JOINT. The shoulder (a ball-and-socket joint) has a greater range of motion than the wrist (a hinge joint), for example.

TEMPERATURE. An increase in either body temperature (as a result of exercise) or external temperature increases range of motion.

PREGNANCY. During pregnancy, a woman's pelvic joints and ligaments are capable of a greater range of motion.

STRETCH SAFELY

Follow these guidelines when you stretch.

✤ If you have a joint or muscle injury, or think you might, consult a doctor before you perform any of these stretches.

✤ Exhale during the stretch phase of the repetition and inhale during the relaxation phase.

✤ During cooldown, choose your stretches based on the stiffness of your muscles, the condition of your joints, and your degree of fatigue. Stretch slowly and gently.

✤ Never force a stretch beyond the point of light discomfort.

✤ You may stretch at any time, not just after a workout. Just warm up your muscles first, whether with a 3-minute walk or a hot bath. *Remember:* Warm up to stretch. *Never* stretch to warm up.

🍀 Breathe deeply when stretching and try to relax into the stretch (avoid tensing your muscles).

🍀 Stretching correctly should feel *good*. You should be able to hold a stretch with a soft smile on your face.

🍀 When doing moving flexibility stretches, begin slowly and increase your speed gradually, as your muscles become warmer and more pliable. Also, be sure to emphasize proper form over speed and number of repetitions.

WARMING UP

Warming up your body before you work out raises your core temperature and increases bloodflow to your muscles, supplying them with the oxygen they need and making them more pliable and ready to work. Warming up also helps to prepare your mind and body for physical exercise. I've designed a warmup routine just for you.

SPORTS-STYLE WARMUP

This 3-minute warmup incorporates the strength and moving flexibility moves in this section. You may repeat it if your muscles do not feel sufficiently supple after the first run-through.

1. March in place. Reach your arms overhead with each inhalation; lower them on the exhalation. Repeat 2 or 3 times.

2. Perform 10 alternating One-Arm Round Front stretches (page 29).

3. Perform 20 alternating Walking Quadriceps stretches (page 40).

4. Perform 15 to 20 Squats (page 166). (*Note:* For the first few repetitions, perform half the range of motion. If possible, increase to the full range of motion by the last repetition.) For the first 5 repetitions, keep your hands on your hips. For the next 5 to 10 repetitions, use your arms: Lower them to your sides in the Squat, then lift them over your head as you return to the starting position. For the last 5 repetitions, add alternating twists: As you stand and extend your arms over your head, twist your body to the right. On the next repetition, twist your body to the left.

5. Perform 10 to 20 Kneeling Lunges (page 25). (*Note:* For the first few repetitions, perform half the range of motion. If possible, increase to the full range of motion by the last repetition.)

6. Pretend to jump rope, mimicking the arm and leg motions. Perform 20 jumps. Start small and enlarge your jumps and arm movements with each repetition.

7. Perform 10 alternating repetitions of the Lunge with One-Arm Reach (page 43).

8. Perform 10 Open-Arm stretches (page 41).

9. Stand in place and take 2 deep breaths, sweeping your arms out to the side and over your head on the inhalation, lowering them with the exhalation.

YOGA-STYLE WARMUP

This 3-minute warmup, for those at the Skilled or Master fitness level, connects breath with movement. The idea is to connect the flow of your body with the flow of your breathing. Avoid stopping in any pose except for Downward-Facing Dog (step 6). Breathe deeply and rhythmically through your nose.

1. Stand with your feet hip-width apart. Inhale and extend your arms over your head, then exhale and lower them. Repeat 2 times.

2. As you continue to breathe, bend your knees and lower yourself into a squat—as if you were going to sit in a chair—as you raise your arms over your head. You are now in the Chair Pose (page 33).

3. Exhale and lower your head and arms toward the floor. Place your palms flat on the floor, if you can, and straighten your legs. You are now in the Standing Forward Bend (page 33). Inhale, then exhale, feeling the stretch in the back of your thighs.

4. Inhale, then exhale. With your hands still on the floor, walk first your right foot and then your left foot backward until your legs are straight. You should look like you are at the top of a pushup. You are now in the Front Plank (page 90).

5. Inhale as you lower your body toward the floor, keeping your elbows close to your sides.

6. Exhale as you push your body back up. (If you cannot perform a full pushup, lower your knees to the floor.) Instead of rising into the Front Plank, push your hips toward the ceiling, leaving your hands flat on the floor. Your body should form an upside-down V, with your tailbone as the point. Check your form: hands flat on the floor with fingers spread open, arms straight with your shoulders away from your ears, long spine with your tailbone lifted toward the ceiling, legs as straight as you can get them (though a slight bend in the knees is okay if your hamstrings feel too much stretch), and heels pressing downward toward the floor.

7. Hold this position for 3 to 5 deep breaths. Focus on form: Keep your weight on your index fingers and thumbs, push your shoulders away from your ears, lift your tailbone to the ceiling, and push your heels into the floor.

8. On the last exhalation in Downward-Facing Dog, step forward first with your right foot and then with your left foot to meet your hands. You are back in the Standing Forward Bend.

9. Inhale, bend your knees, and raise your torso so that you are back in the Chair Pose.

10. Exhale and stand up straight. Repeat the warmup 2 more times.

COOLING DOWN

You want to cool down after a workout to avoid having blood pool in your limbs and waste (like lactic acid) build up in your muscles, and to lessen muscle soreness and stiffness.

I've suggested several cooldown routines below. Perform the one of your choice at the end of each workout.

COOLDOWN 1 (STATIC STRETCHES ONLY)

1. One-Arm Round Front

2. Standing Quadriceps

3. Kneeling Lunge (static version)

4. Modified Hurdler

5. Seated Forward Bend

6. Cobra Pose

7. Child's Pose with Reach Across (static version)

8. Spinal Twist

9. Reaching Butterfly

COOLDOWN 2 (MOVING FLEXIBILITY STRETCHES ONLY)

1. Walking Quadriceps

2. Lunge with One-Arm Reach

3. Single-Arm Reach Back

4. Chair to Standing Forward Bend

5. Bent-Arm Overhead

6. Single-Arm Reach Across (moving flexibility version)

7. Lying Split Leg

8. Child's Pose to Upward-Facing Dog

9. Open Arm

COOLDOWN 3 (STATIC AND MOVING FLEXIBILITY STRETCHES)

1. Walking Quadriceps

2. One-Arm Round Front

3. Kneeling Lunge (moving flexibility version)

4. Open Arm

5. Seated Forward Bend

6. Reaching Butterfly

7. Single-Arm Reach Back

8. Bent-Arm Overhead

9. Child's Pose with Reach Across (moving flexibility version)

TANK TOP
Arms

There's something alluring about women with sleek, toned arms—sculpted shoulders, fit biceps with a hint of muscle, and tight, firm triceps (the back of the upper arm). Tank tops and strapless dresses were made for beautiful arms, which display both strength and femininity.

Building firm, rounded shoulders with strength training can make the waistline look smaller. Full biceps give arms a pleasing, feminine curve. And although the triceps make up about two-thirds of the entire arm, they are used less often in everyday life than the biceps, so you've got to put them to work to keep the wiggles and jiggles away.

In 4 weeks or less, the moves in this section will define your shoulders, firm your biceps, and tighten your triceps so they don't wave good-bye when you do.

NOVICE

FRONT RAISE

SHOULDER PRESS

TRICEPS KICKBACK

LYING TRICEPS EXTENSION

BICEPS CURL

HAMMER CURL

CHEST PRESS

MODIFIED PUSHUP

SKILLED

LATERAL RAISE

REAR DELTOID FLY

MODIFIED PLANK

OVERHEAD TRICEPS EXTENSION

TRICEPS DIP

ROTATIONAL SHOULDER PRESS

CONCENTRATION CURL

CHEST FLY

MASTER

PLANK HOLD WALKOUT

YOGI PUSHUP

ONE-ARM TRICEPS PUSHUP

FRONT TO SIDE PLANK

BENT-OVER ROW

SIDE PLANK WITH ARM RAISE

ARNOLD PRESS

SHOULDER SHIMMY

PART 1

TANK TOP
Arms

There's something alluring about women with sleek, toned arms—sculpted shoulders, fit biceps with a hint of muscle, and tight, firm triceps (the back of the upper arm). Tank tops and strapless dresses were made for beautiful arms, which display both strength and femininity.

Building firm, rounded shoulders with strength training can make the waistline look smaller. Full biceps give arms a pleasing, feminine curve. And although the triceps make up about two-thirds of the entire arm, they are used less often in everyday life than the biceps, so you've got to put them to work to keep the wiggles and jiggles away.

In 4 weeks or less, the moves in this section will define your shoulders, firm your biceps, and tighten your triceps so they don't wave good-bye when you do.

NOVICE	SKILLED	MASTER
FRONT RAISE	LATERAL RAISE	PLANK HOLD WALKOUT
SHOULDER PRESS	REAR DELTOID FLY	YOGI PUSHUP
TRICEPS KICKBACK	MODIFIED PLANK	ONE-ARM TRICEPS PUSHUP
LYING TRICEPS EXTENSION	OVERHEAD TRICEPS EXTENSION	FRONT TO SIDE PLANK
BICEPS CURL	TRICEPS DIP	BENT-OVER ROW
HAMMER CURL	ROTATIONAL SHOULDER PRESS	SIDE PLANK WITH ARM RAISE
CHEST PRESS	CONCENTRATION CURL	ARNOLD PRESS
MODIFIED PUSHUP	CHEST FLY	SHOULDER SHIMMY

1

TANK TOP ARMS
NOVICE

If you're new to strength training, these moves for the upper body—the shoulders, biceps, and triceps—are for you. As a beginner, you'll focus on proper form and technique, so follow my step-by-step instructions to the letter. If you have joined a gym, bring this book along and set it on the floor beside you. (Ask the trainers for help, too—that's why they're around.) If you are working out at home, you'll need a set of dumbbells. A Bosu ball and/or a stability ball are optional for use if you wish to try the variations in the "At the Gym" sections. Consider investing in an inexpensive full-length mirror, too, so you can continually check your form.

FEATURED EXERCISES:
♣FRONT RAISE
♣SHOULDER PRESS
♣TRICEPS KICKBACK
♣LYING TRICEPS EXTENSION
♣BICEPS CURL
♣HAMMER CURL
♣CHEST PRESS
♣MODIFIED PUSHUP

FRONT RAISE

This move tones the front of the shoulders (anterior deltoids),
helping design sleek, sexy shoulders—a must for tank tops.

SETS AND REPS

BEGINNER: 1 to 2 sets,
8 to 12 repetitions,
3- to 5-pound dumbbells
INTERMEDIATE: 2 to 3 sets,
8 to 12 repetitions,
5- to 10-pound dumbbells
ADVANCED: 3 sets, 8 to 12 repetitions,
8- to 15-pound dumbbells

STARTING POSITION

Stand with your feet hip-width apart and
your knees slightly bent, holding the
dumbbells horizontally in front of your
thighs, palms facing you. Contract your
abdominal muscles, align your hips and
shoulders, and draw your shoulders back
and down.

THE MOVE

Lift the dumbbells, palms down, until your
arms are parallel with the floor. Slowly
lower the dumbbells, returning to the
starting position to complete 1 repetition.

FOCUS ON FORM

✤ Contract your abdominals throughout
  the move.
✤ Keep your arms straight, but avoid
  locking your elbows.
✤ Lower the dumbbells slowly for
  maximum resistance.
✤ Keep your shoulders down and away
  from your ears. If they shrug upward
  and your head moves forward, you are
  lifting too much weight.

AT HOME/AT THE GYM

AT HOME: Assume the starting position,
but perform the move with your hands in
the supinated position (palms facing forward). You'll find that it's harder to shrug
your shoulders.

AT THE GYM: Try this move as you stand
on a Bosu ball or sit on a stability ball.
These variations will challenge your balance, so use lighter dumbbells at first.

BEGINNER

If lifting both dumbbells at the same time
fatigues your shoulders, alternate arms:
Lift one arm only and, as you return to
the starting position, start to lift the other
arm. For additional back support, sit as
you perform the move.

INTERMEDIATE

Perform the first step of the move, but
don't lower the dumbbells. Instead, extend
your arms out to the sides at shoulder
height, then lower them to your sides.
Move the dumbbells to the front of your
thighs and repeat.

ADVANCED

Immediately after this move, perform
1 Shoulder Press (see page 56). Hold the
dumbbells in front of your thighs, but
don't straighten your arms. Instead, bend
your elbows and, keeping the dumbbells
close to your body, use your shoulders to
lift the dumbbells above your head. Lower
the dumbbells and repeat until you complete 1 set.

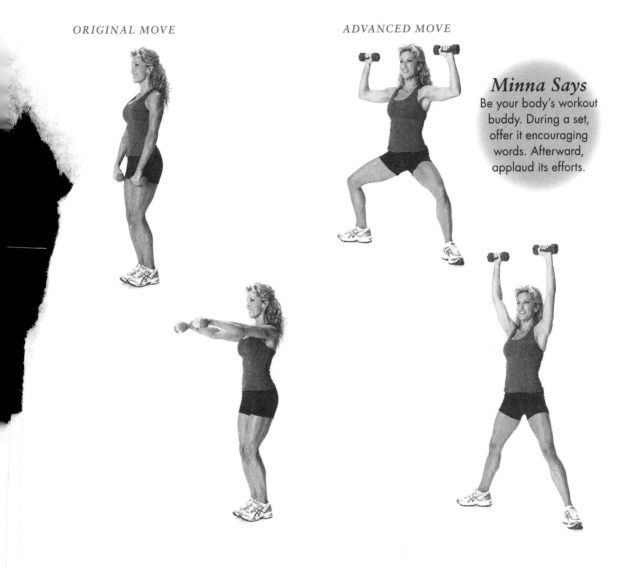

Minna Says
Be your body's workout buddy. During a set, offer it encouraging words. Afterward, applaud its efforts.

USE YOUR HEAD
Imagine you are lifting a sheet upward in front of your body, as if to shake out the wrinkles.

BREATHWORK
Exhale as you lift the dumbbells. Inhale as you slowly lower them.

SUGGESTED STRETCH
Moving Flexibility:
Single-Arm Reach Across
(page 37)

SHOULDER PRESS

This move strengthens and shapes the anterior deltoids,
keeping you in sleek, sculpted "summer shoulders" all year-round.

SETS AND REPS

BEGINNER: 1 to 2 sets,
8 to 12 repetitions,
3- to 5-pound dumbbells
INTERMEDIATE: 2 to 3 sets,
8 to 12 repetitions,
8- to 12-pound dumbbells
ADVANCED: 3 sets, 8 to 12 repetitions,
10- to 20-pound dumbbells

STARTING POSITION

Sit on a sturdy chair or bench. Contract
your abdominal muscles and draw your
shoulders back and down. With your arms
bent at shoulder level, hold the dumbbells
to the sides of your head, aligning your
elbows directly beneath your wrists with
your palms facing forward.

THE MOVE

Raise the dumbbells until your arms are
over your head. Slowly lower the dumbbells to the starting position to complete
1 repetition.

FOCUS ON FORM

✤ Contract your abdominals throughout
   the move.
✤ Keep your shoulders down and away
   from your ears.
✤ Raise and lower the dumbbells slowly,
   with control.

AT HOME/AT THE GYM

AT HOME: Perform external rotations with
2- to 5-pound dumbbells. Assume the
starting position. Keeping your upper arms
immobile, rotate your arms forward
90 degrees and lower the dumbbells until
your hands are parallel with the floor.
Then, rotate your arms, lifting the dumbbells to the starting position. Repeat until
you complete 1 set.

AT THE GYM: Beginners, try this move on
the seated shoulder press machine—it will
help you learn the proper form. Ask a
trainer to help you adjust the machine to
your height. Intermediate and advanced
readers, try this move while sitting on a
stability ball.

BEGINNER

Concentrate on perfecting your form.
Progress to heavier dumbbells only when
you have mastered the move.

INTERMEDIATE

Perform this move in a standing position.
Bend your knees slightly and contract
your abdominals throughout.

ADVANCED

Combine this move with the Plié Squat
(see page 192) while holding two dumbbells. Perform the squat first and, as you
rise, perform this move.

ORIGINAL MOVE   ADVANCED MOVE

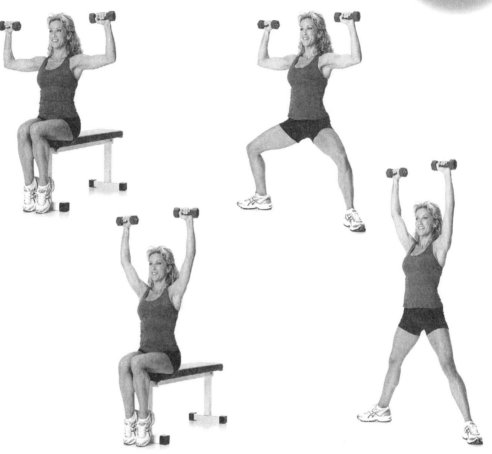

USE YOUR HEAD

Keeping your shoulders away from your ears can help prevent injury. To help you remember this, picture a string tied to each shoulder. As you raise the dumbbells, the string pulls your shoulders down.

BREATHWORK

Exhale as you press the dumbbells over your head. Inhale as you lower them.

SUGGESTED STRETCH

Moving Flexibility:
Open Arm
(page 41)

TRICEPS KICKBACK

This move strengthens the triceps, eliminating the dreaded upper-arm wiggle and jiggle.

SETS AND REPS

BEGINNER: 1 to 2 sets,
8 to 12 repetitions per side,
3- to 5-pound dumbbells
INTERMEDIATE: 2 to 3 sets,
8 to 12 repetitions per side,
5- to 10-pound dumbbells
ADVANCED: 3 sets,
8 to 12 repetitions per side,
10- to 15-pound dumbbells

STARTING POSITION

Stand with your feet hip-width apart. Hold a dumbbell in your left hand, with your arm hanging at your side and your palm facing inward. Contract your abdominal muscles, align your shoulders and hips, and draw your shoulders back and down. With your left foot, take a big step backward so that your feet are staggered 2 to 3 feet apart. Bend your right knee, place your right hand on your right thigh, and lean forward, keeping your back straight. Bend your left arm at the elbow and hold the dumbbell close to your body. Your elbow should point backward and your knuckles should point toward the floor.

THE MOVE

From the starting position, straighten your left arm as you extend it behind you. Bend your elbow and slowly lower the dumbbell to the starting position. Complete 8 to 12 repetitions, and then switch your foot and arm positions and do 8 to 12 repetitions with your right arm to complete 1 set.

FOCUS ON FORM

♣ Keep your upper arm motionless. Only your forearm should move, swinging slowly back and forth at the elbow, like a hinge.
♣ Keep your back straight and lean forward from your hips.
♣ Relax your shoulders. If they hunch up, you are lifting too much weight.
♣ Contract your abdominals throughout.

AT HOME/AT THE GYM

AT HOME: If you own exercise bands, perform the move below. Otherwise, perform the move as directed above.
AT THE GYM: Try this move with an exercise band. Step on one end of the band so that it comes up on the inside of your foot, and grasp the handle. Perform the move as described above.

BEGINNER

If your back or legs tire in the standing position, kneel on the floor or on a mat, lean forward, and perform the move.

INTERMEDIATE

Try performing the move with both arms at the same time and feet together.

ADVANCED

Try all three palm positions to target all three heads of your triceps. After performing 1 set of the basic move, try 1 set with your palms facing backward and another with your palms facing foward.

ORIGINAL MOVE

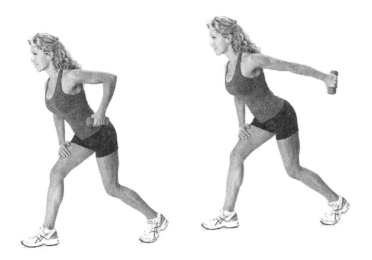

INTERMEDIATE MOVE

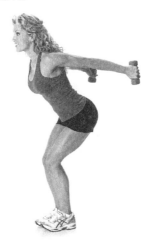

ADVANCED MOVE

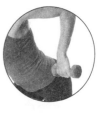

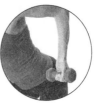

USE YOUR HEAD

Imagine that you work on an assembly line and that your job is to move your "product"—your lower arm, hand, and dumbbell—from point A to point B.

BREATHWORK

Exhale as you straighten your arm. Inhale as you return it to the starting position.

SUGGESTED STRETCH
Moving Flexibility:
Bent-Arm Overhead
(page 38)

LYING TRICEPS EXTENSION

Master this move, which shapes and tones the triceps, and you'll be rewarded with taut, toned upper arms.

SETS AND REPS

BEGINNER: 1 to 2 sets,
8 to 12 repetitions,
5- to 8-pound dumbbell
INTERMEDIATE: 2 to 3 sets,
8 to 12 repetitions,
8- to 12-pound dumbbell
ADVANCED: 3 sets,
8 to 12 repetitions,
10- to 20-pound dumbbell

STARTING POSITION

Lie on your back on a bench. If you're working out at home, lie on the floor or on a mat. Hold the dumbbell vertically with both hands, with your palm against the inside of the upper end and your hand cupping the weight. Your thumbs and index fingers should meet to create a heart shape. Bend your knees and place your feet flat on the bench or floor. Contract your abdominal muscles. Lift the dumbbell over your head so that the end that you're *not* grasping is closest to and slightly behind your head.

THE MOVE

Keeping your upper arms still and bending only your elbows, lower the dumbbell behind your head. Fully stretch your triceps at the bottom of the move. Squeeze your triceps to return the dumbbell to the starting position to complete 1 repetition.

FOCUS ON FORM

♣ Keep your elbows close together. Flaring them out to the sides lessens the effort for your triceps.
♣ Keep your upper arms still. Only your forearms should move down and up.
♣ Contract your abdominals throughout the move to protect your lower back.

AT HOME/AT THE GYM

AT HOME: Perform the move as directed above. If you own a stability ball, perform the move below.
AT THE GYM: Try this move with a stability ball: Lie with your upper back on the ball and your pelvis hanging off of it. Perform the move.

BEGINNER

If you feel this move too much in your back muscles, make sure you are not moving your upper arms. If you still feel a strain, replace the move with the Overhead Triceps Extension (see page 78).

INTERMEDIATE

Try using a heavier dumbbell to perform the move. Lower it to the level of your ears rather than behind your head.

ADVANCED

Follow every set of extensions with a set of triceps presses. Keep the dumbbell above the level of your head. Then, draw it toward your chest. Touch the dumbbell lightly to your chest, then press it straight upward, keeping your wrists directly over the midline of your chest.

Minna Says

To reshape your body, you must first reshape your mind. Banish negative self-talk that works against your efforts, and replace it with positive thoughts.

ORIGINAL MOVE

ADVANCED MOVE

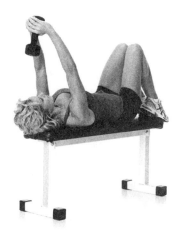

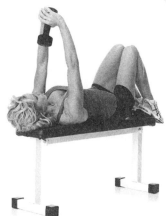

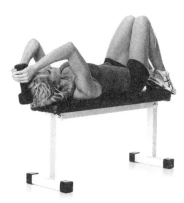

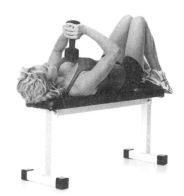

USE YOUR HEAD

Some fitness buffs call Lying Triceps Extensions "skullcrushers," and for a good reason: As you lower the dumbbell, you can conk yourself in the head if you aren't concentrating on controlling its weight. Stay focused!

BREATHWORK

Inhale as you lower the dumbbell. Exhale as you return to the starting position.

BICEPS CURL

This move builds beautiful, bodacious arms by sculpting and strengthening the muscle on the front of your upper arm (the biceps).

SETS AND REPS

BEGINNER: 1 to 2 sets,
8 to 12 repetitions per side,
3- to 8-pound dumbbells
INTERMEDIATE: 2 to 3 sets,
8 to 12 repetitions per side,
5- to 10-pound dumbbells
ADVANCED: 3 sets,
8 to 12 repetitions per side,
8- to 15-pound dumbbells

STARTING POSITION

Stand with your together, holding the dumbbells at your sides with your palms facing inward. Bend your knees slightly. Contract your abdominal muscles, align your shoulders and hips, and draw your shoulders down and back.

THE MOVE

Start with your left arm. Raise the dumbbell toward your shoulder. When the dumbbell reaches hip level, rotate it so that your palm faces upward. Slowly lower the dumbbell and repeat with your right arm. Continue, alternating repetitions, until you complete 1 set.

Minna Says

To rev up your motivation, write your top three fitness goals on an index card and tape the card where you'll see it during your workout. Then achieve them one by one.

FOCUS ON FORM

✤ Immobilize your upper arm by tucking your elbow into your side. Avoid raising your elbow as you lift the dumbbell.
✤ Maintain erect posture. Leaning backward places stress on the lower back.
✤ To avoid forearm fatigue, maintain a relaxed grip on the dumbbells and align your wrists with your forearms.
✤ Lift the dumbbells slowly, in a controlled, fluid manner. If you're swinging and jerking as you raise them, you are lifting too much weight.

AT HOME/AT THE GYM

AT HOME: Try a side curl. Assume the starting position described above, but when you raise the dumbbell to hip level, turn your arm as much as possible so that your palm faces outward. As you curl the dumbbell, lift your arm out to the side like a wing.

AT THE GYM: Sit on an incline bench. Hold the dumbbells at your sides with your palms facing inward. Perform the move, keeping your upper arms still.

BEGINNER

Focus on keeping your upper arms still as you perform the move. As you lift each dumbbell, your elbow should point toward the floor.

INTERMEDIATE

Do not rest between repetitions. When your left arm is halfway back to the starting position, begin to lift the dumbbell in your right hand.

ADVANCED

Assume the basic starting position, but curl both arms at the same time. Keep your back straight and your upper arms still.

ORIGINAL MOVE

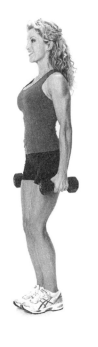 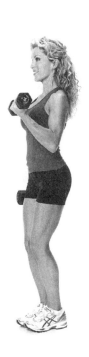

ADVANCED MOVE

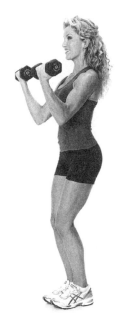

USE YOUR HEAD

Imagine that your biceps are little loaves of bread baking in the oven. Each time you lift a dumbbell, imagine the loaf rising and filling out.

BREATHWORK

Exhale as you curl the dumbbell upward. Inhale as you lower it.

SUGGESTED STRETCH

Moving Flexibility:
Single-Arm Reach Back
(page 39)

HAMMER CURL

This move sculpts the biceps, strengthens the forearm, and targets the brachialis, the muscle that runs along the outside of the upper arm, adding gorgeous shape and definition.

SETS AND REPS

BEGINNER: 1 to 2 sets,
16 to 24 alternating repetitions,
3- to 8-pound dumbbells
INTERMEDIATE: 2 to 3 sets,
16 to 24 alternating repetitions,
8- to 12-pound dumbbells
ADVANCED: 3 sets,
16 to 24 alternating repetitions,
10- to 20-pound dumbbells

STARTING POSITION

Grasp a dumbbell in each hand. Stand with your feet together and your arms at your sides with your palms facing inward. Bend your knees slightly, contract your abdominal muscles, align your shoulders and hips, and draw your shoulders back and down.

THE MOVE

Slowly curl the dumbbell in your left hand toward the front of your shoulder, using only your biceps. Keep your wrist turned so that your palm faces inward, toward your body, throughout the move. Slowly lower the dumbbell to the starting position. Keep a slight bend in your elbow at the bottom of the movement. Repeat, alternating repetitions with the left and right arms, until you complete 1 set.

Minna Says
Failure is real only if we give up. We all get knocked down. What matters is that we get up again.

FOCUS ON FORM

❖ Avoid rocking forward. Lower the dumbbells slowly and with control.
❖ Keep your elbows at your sides throughout the move. Flaring them out or moving them forward or backward reduces the move's effectiveness.
❖ To avoid tiring your forearms, immobilize your wrists and maintain a relaxed grip on the dumbbells.
❖ Move your forearms only. Swinging your arms will take the workload off your biceps.
❖ Contract your abdominals throughout the move to support your lower back.

AT HOME/AT THE GYM

AT HOME: Try a reverse curl. Assume the starting position, but turn your wrists so that your palms face backward. Perform the move. Repeat until you complete the set of alternating movements.
AT THE GYM: Perform this move on the cable crossover machine. Attach the ropes to the lower cable. Adjust the machine to the desired amount of weight. Grip the ropes near the wooden balls. Stand facing the cable. Assume the basic starting position and perform the move, using both arms at once.

BEGINNER

If your lower back gets tired, sit on a chair or bench to perform the move.

INTERMEDIATE

Do not rest between repetitions. When your left arm is halfway back to the starting position, begin to lift the dumbbell in your right hand.

ADVANCED

Perform the move with one foot off the floor. Assume the basic starting position. Lift one foot off the floor as far as is comfortable, depending on your strength and flexibility, keeping both legs and your back straight. Perform the move; halfway through each set, switch legs.

ORIGINAL MOVE

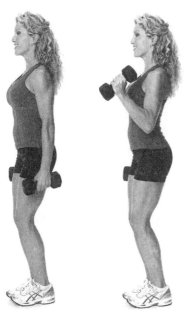

ADVANCED MOVE

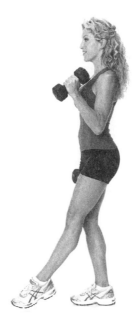

USE YOUR HEAD

As you perform this move, imagine driving a nail into a board in slow motion. To lift your arm, contract your biceps muscle hard as you lift the hammer. Then lower your arm as if you are precisely targeting the head of the nail.

BREATHWORK

Exhale as you lift the dumbbell. Inhale as you lower it.

SUGGESTED STRETCH

Moving Flexibility:
Single-Arm Reach Back
(page 39)

♣ CHEST PRESS

This classic move is a mainstay for a fit, strong upper body.
It defines and tones the chest, shoulders, and triceps.

SETS AND REPS

BEGINNER: 1 to 2 sets,
8 to 12 repetitions,
5- to 8-pound dumbbells
INTERMEDIATE: 2 to 3 sets,
8 to 12 repetitions,
8- to 12-pound dumbbells
ADVANCED: 3 sets,
8 to 12 repetitions,
12- to 20-pound dumbbells

STARTING POSITION

Lie on your back on the floor with your knees bent and your feet flat on the floor, holding the dumbbells at your sides with your palms facing downward. Contract your abdominal muscles and lift the dumbbells over your head and toward the ceiling, keeping your thumbs pointing toward each other. Draw your shoulders back and down.

THE MOVE

Bend your elbows and lower the dumbbells until your upper arms are parallel with the floor. Position your wrists directly over your elbows. Using your chest, shoulder, and triceps muscles, return the dumbbells to the starting position. Repeat until you complete 1 set.

Minna Says
When we think we know all there is to know about our bodies, we stop seeing results. When you strive to improve, your body shows it.

FOCUS ON FORM

♣ You must draw your shoulders back and down. This small movement places more of the workload on your chest muscles and helps prevent shoulder injury.

♣ Contract your abdominals throughout the move.

AT HOME/AT THE GYM

AT HOME: Intermediate or advanced readers only, if you own a stability ball, try the move below. If you don't own a stability ball or you're a beginner, perform the move as described above.

AT THE GYM: Beginners, try this move on the seated chest press machine to learn the proper range of motion. Have a trainer adjust the machine to your height. Select the desired amount of weight. While holding the bars, press the weight forward, then bend your elbows and resist the weight as you return to the starting position. Intermediate and advanced readers, perform the move on a stability ball. Lie faceup with your shoulders and neck on the ball, knees bent, and feet flat on the floor. Contract your abdominals, raise the dumbbells over your head (with your wrists directly over your shoulders), and perform the move.

BEGINNER

Focus on form, particularly on keeping your shoulders back and down as you press.

INTERMEDIATE

This challenging variation requires a chair. Assume the basic starting position, but place your lower legs on the seat of a chair, aligning your knees directly over your hips. Raise the dumbbells over your head. Continue to hold your left arm over your head as you bend your right elbow and lower the dumbbell until your elbow just touches the floor. Press the dumbbell upward, hold it over your head, then lower your left arm. Repeat, alternating sides, until you complete 1 set.

ADVANCED

Alternate repetitions of the Chest Press and Chest Fly (see page 86). For a major challenge, bend your knees to 90 degrees, so that your lower legs are parallel to the floor. (It's the same leg position described above but without the chair.) Alternate repetitions of the Chest Press and Chest Fly until you complete 1 set.

ORIGINAL MOVE

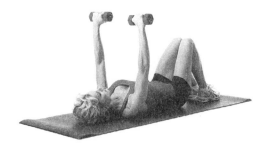

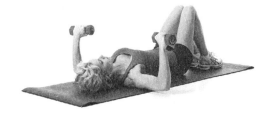

ADVANCED MOVE

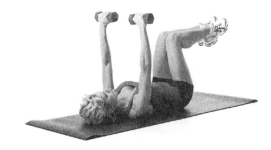

USE YOUR HEAD

Think of trying to push open a very heavy door as someone is holding your shoulders and trying to pull you away. Contract your chest, shoulder, and triceps muscles— hard—and make them burn as you slowly but surely push open that door.

BREATHWORK

Exhale as you press the dumbbells over your head. Inhale as you return them to the starting position.

SUGGESTED STRETCH

Moving Flexibility:
Open Arm
(page 41)

♣ MODIFIED PUSHUP

This "boot camp" move builds power, stamina—and a toned, taut upper body. You'll benefit from toned and strengthened arm, abdominal, and chest muscles and more defined shoulders and triceps.

SETS AND REPS

BEGINNER: 1 to 2 sets, 8 to 15 repetitions, or as many as you can perform with good form

INTERMEDIATE: 2 to 3 sets, 8 to 15 repetitions

ADVANCED: 3 sets, 8 to 15 repetitions, combined with full pushups (see below)

STARTING POSITION

Get down on all fours, positioning your wrists directly beneath your shoulders. Extend your legs behind you, supporting yourself on your knees, so that your body makes one long, straight line from your head to your knees. Contract your abdominal muscles.

THE MOVE

Bending your elbows, lower your body until just before it touches the floor. Using your chest, shoulder, and triceps muscles, return to the starting position.

FOCUS ON FORM

♣ Contract your abdominals throughout the move to keep your back straight (avoid sagging or rounding).

♣ As you push up, avoid locking your elbows. Keep them soft at the top of the move.

♣ Keep your shoulders down and away from your ears.

AT HOME/AT THE GYM

AT HOME: After the last repetition of a set, try holding the top of the move (the full Front Plank; see page 90) for 10 to 30 seconds.

AT THE GYM: Try the seated chest press machine. Adjust the machine to fit your height, and ask a trainer to help you line up its points with your joints. Add the desired amount of weight. Press the weight forward, then return to the starting position.

BEGINNER

To make the move less challenging, bring your knees closer to your body, directly beneath your hips.

INTERMEDIATE

Get low, go slow, and push up with power. Lower your body on a count of three, then push up on a count of one.

ADVANCED

Try a combo of full and Modified Pushups. Perform as many full pushups as you can with good form, then continue with Modified Pushups. To perform a full pushup, assume the same upper body position as the modified version but extend your legs straight back, supporting yourself on your toes.

ORIGINAL MOVE

ADVANCED MOVE

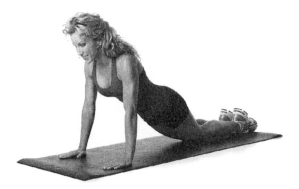

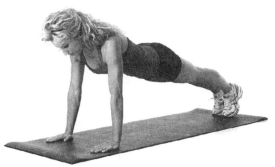

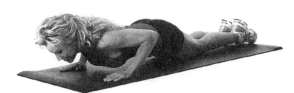

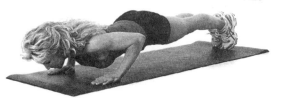

USE YOUR HEAD

Think of an athlete you admire (my list includes Florence Griffith Joyner, Mary Lou Retton, Marion Jones, and Serena Williams) and how she has challenged her body to its limit. As you perform each repetition, feel your muscles striving to achieve their potential.

BREATHWORK

Inhale as you lower your body. Exhale as you return to the starting position.

SUGGESTED STRETCH
Moving Flexibility:
Open Arm
(page 41)

2

TANK TOP ARMS
SKILLED

If you've mastered the Novice exercises, or have been working out with weights for at least 6 months, performing these moves will take your upper body to the next level. They focus on strength, flexibility, and balance and further challenge your core musculature. If you are working out at home, you will need a set of dumbbells. A Bosu ball and/or a medicine ball are optional for use if you want to perform the variations in the "At the Gym" sections.

FEATURED EXERCISES:

♣LATERAL RAISE

♣REAR DELTOID FLY

♣MODIFIED PLANK

♣OVERHEAD TRICEPS EXTENSION

♣TRICEPS DIP

♣ROTATIONAL SHOULDER PRESS

♣CONCENTRATION CURL

♣CHEST FLY

LATERAL RAISE

This move gives the sides of the shoulders an appealing roundness—perfect for sleeveless tops and summer dresses.

SETS AND REPS

BEGINNER: 1 to 2 sets,
8 to 12 repetitions,
3- to 5-pound dumbbells
INTERMEDIATE: 2 to 3 sets,
8 to 12 repetitions,
5- to 8-pound dumbbells
ADVANCED: 3 sets, 8 to 12 repetitions,
8- to 15-pound dumbbells

STARTING POSITION

Stand with your feet together, knees slightly bent, holding the dumbbells at your sides with your palms facing inward. Keep your hips and shoulders level and aligned and your shoulders drawn back and down. Contract your abdominal muscles. Tilt slightly forward from the waist.

THE MOVE

With your elbows slightly bent, raise your upper arms out to the side, like wings, until your elbows reach shoulder height. Slowly lower the dumbbells to the starting position to complete 1 repetition. Repeat until you complete 1 set.

Minna Says
We feel best when our homes are clean, organized, and comfortable. The body—the home of the spirit—deserves the same attention and treatment.

FOCUS ON FORM

❖ Contract your abdominals throughout the move to support your lower back.
❖ As you lift your arms, your palms should face the floor. Avoid rotating your arms backward to try to lift the weight, because this may injure your rotator cuff.
❖ Avoid clunking the dumbbells together at the bottom of the move—it may lead to injury.
❖ Keep your shoulders down and away from your ears. Shrugging them will create tension in your neck and shoulders.

AT HOME/AT THE GYM

AT HOME: Perform this move as described above.
AT THE GYM: Try this move on the lower pulley of the cable crossover machine, one arm at a time. Attach a handlebar to the lower pulley and select the desired weight. Stand with your right side next to the pulley and hold the handle with your left hand in front of your body. Keeping your arm straight, raise it up to the side, then lower it to the starting position. Complete 1 set, then switch sides.

BEGINNER

If you're feeling this move in muscles other than your deltoids (the sides of your shoulders), try sitting on a sturdy chair and holding the dumbbells at your sides, or try bending your elbows to 90 degrees. Raise your arms, leading with your elbows, until your elbows are at shoulder height.

INTERMEDIATE

Try a one-armed version of this move. Lie on one side with your feet flat on the floor and 1 to 2 feet apart for stability. Support your head with the hand of your bottom arm. Grasp the dumbbell with the other hand, palm facing down. Raise the dumbbell into the air until your arm is straight up. Slowly lower it and repeat until you complete 1 set.

ADVANCED

Try a drop set: For each set, use dumbbells of a different weight—heavy, medium, and light. Begin with the heaviest set of dumbbells, performing as many repetitions as you can with good form (8 to 12 repetitions). Without pausing, repeat with the medium and then the light dumbbells, again performing as many repetitions as you can while maintaining form.

ORIGINAL MOVE

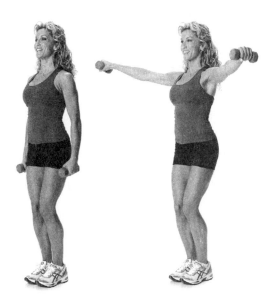

INTERMEDIATE MOVE

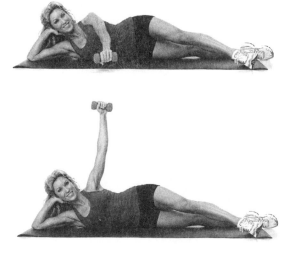

USE YOUR HEAD

As you extend your arms outward and away from your body, really lengthen and elongate them, as a ballerina would. Also remember to squeeze your shoulder blades together to keep your shoulders back and down.

BREATHWORK

Exhale as you raise the dumbbells. Inhale as you lower them.

SUGGESTED STRETCH
Moving Flexibility:
Single-Arm Reach Across
(page 37)

♣ REAR DELTOID FLY

This move helps build shoulders you'll dare to bare by sculpting and strengthening the backs of the shoulders (the posterior deltoids).

SETS AND REPS

BEGINNER: 1 to 2 sets,
8 to 12 repetitions,
2- to 3-pound dumbbells
INTERMEDIATE: 2 to 3 sets,
8 to 12 repetitions,
5- to 8-pound dumbbells
ADVANCED: 3 sets,
8 to 12 repetitions,
8- to 12-pound dumbbells

STARTING POSITION

Stand with your feet together or, for greater stability, with one foot 2 to 3 feet in front of the other. Bend your knees slightly and tilt your torso forward 45 degrees. Hold the dumbbells in front of your thighs with your thumbs pointing at each other and your arms straight. Contract your abdominal muscles and draw your shoulders back and down.

THE MOVE

Slowly lift the dumbbells out to the sides until your arms are parallel with the floor. Keep your arms straight, but avoid locking your elbows. Lower the dumbbells slowly to complete 1 repetition. Repeat until you finish 1 set.

Minna Says

Feeling down? Stand tall. Good posture can boost your confidence in an instant.

FOCUS ON FORM

✤ Contract your abdominals throughout the move to support your lower back.
✤ Keep your shoulders relaxed and away from your ears.
✤ Lower the dumbbells until they are directly beneath your shoulders. Do not touch them together at the bottom of the move.

AT HOME/AT THE GYM

AT HOME: Try this move on the floor, without dumbbells. Lie on your belly with your arms extended straight out at shoulder height, palms flat on the floor. Lift your arms off the floor as high as you can without tensing your shoulders. Lower your arms and repeat.
AT THE GYM: Lie with your abdomen on a stability ball and your upper body hanging slightly off the ball. Lift your arms until they are parallel with the floor. Lower your arms and repeat.

BEGINNER

Perform this move while sitting on a sturdy chair or bench. Lean forward until your chest touches or almost touches your upper thighs. If your upper back becomes extremely fatigued, increase the bend in your elbows.

INTERMEDIATE

Combine this move with the Bent-Over Row (see page 98). Holding the dumbbell in your right hand, place your left foot in front of your right. Bend your right elbow slightly and, squeezing your shoulder blades together, lift your arm out to the side until your upper arm is parallel with the floor. Lower the dumbbell, then immediately perform the Rear Deltoid Fly by lifting your right arm straight up and out to the side until it is parallel with the floor, then return to the starting position. Continue to alternate between the moves for 1 set, then switch sides. If you're performing an odd number of sets, switch sides halfway through each set.

ADVANCED

Try this move with the Side Plank hold (see page 96). Holding a dumbbell in your left hand, assume the Side Plank position, with your right hand on the floor. Lift your left arm, keeping your thumb down, until your left arm is straight up and aligned with your right arm. Lower your left arm until your hand is about 12 inches off the floor. Avoid twisting your torso—if you do twist, your abdominal muscles will get a better workout than your rear deltoids.

ORIGINAL MOVE

ADVANCED MOVE

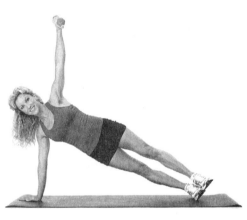

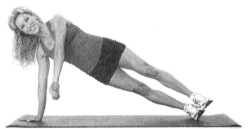

USE YOUR HEAD
Imagine that you are an eagle wheeling gracefully through the sky. Lift and lower your "wings" to "fly" as your body remains motionless, as an eagle's does.

BREATHWORK
Exhale as you lift the dumbbells. Inhale as you lower them.

SUGGESTED STRETCH
Static:
Single-Arm Reach Across
(page 26)
Moving Flexibility:
Bent-Arm Overhead (page 38)

MODIFIED PLANK

This move—a classic yoga pose—tightens your core while it whittles your waist. It strengthens the muscles of the core and shoulders, particularly the front and middle deltoids.

SETS AND REPS

BEGINNER: 1 to 2 sets, hold for 10 to 30 seconds
INTERMEDIATE: 2 to 3 sets, hold for 10 to 30 seconds, or shoulder rocks (see opposite page), 12 to 20 alternating repetitions
ADVANCED: 3 sets, hold for 10 to 30 seconds, or arm lifts (see opposite page), 12 to 20 alternating repetitions

STARTING POSITION

Get down on all fours. Lower yourself onto your forearms so that your palms are flat on the floor and your elbows are directly beneath your shoulders. Extend your legs straight back so that only your toes are touching the floor. Contract your abdominal muscles and draw your navel toward your spine. Your body should form one long, straight line from your head to your heels.

THE MOVE

Hold this position for the length of time indicated for your fitness level.

FOCUS ON FORM

♣ Draw your navel toward your spine to maintain the long line of your body.
♣ Align your head with your spine. Avoid drooping or lifting your head to break the line.
♣ Contract your quadriceps muscles (in the front of the thighs) to help you hold the position.

AT HOME/AT THE GYM

AT HOME: Add a hand walk to the move. Assume the starting position as described. Move your right palm to the right side, so that it is in line with your right elbow. Then move your left palm to the left side. Push your body to the top of a pushup position. Return your right forearm to the original position on the right, followed by your left forearm, so that you are once again in the Modified Plank position. Repeat, leading the walk with your right hand for 5 to 8 repetitions, then leading with your left hand for 5 to 8 repetitions.
AT THE GYM: Perform the Modified Plank on the round side of a Bosu ball.

Minna Says
Just when you think you've got to give up, find the last ounce of energy in you and push to cross the finish line.

BEGINNER

If holding the Modified Plank proves too challenging, drop to your knees for a second or two, then return to the move. Work up to holding the position for 10 to 30 seconds.

INTERMEDIATE

Hold the position, then rock gently from side to side. Rock from your shoulders, tilting a few inches to the right, then a few inches to the left. Continue to rock for 12 to 20 repetitions.

ADVANCED

Perform the move, but extend your left arm over your head. Return it to the starting position and repeat with your right arm. Complete 12 to 20 alternating repetitions.

ORIGINAL MOVE

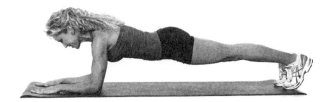

ADVANCED MOVE

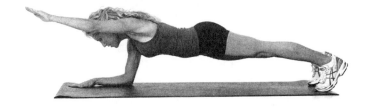

USE YOUR HEAD

Imagine being stretched like a rubber band, with your head being pulled in one direction and your tailbone, legs, and feet in the other. Picture every vertebra in your back opening up . . . *ahh!*

BREATHWORK

Breathe deeply and rhythmically through your nose, pulling the air against the back of your throat.

SUGGESTED STRETCH

Static:
Single-Arm Reach Across
(page 26)

OVERHEAD TRICEPS EXTENSION

This move busts "bat wings" so you can wear your tank tops with pride. It shapes and tones the triceps.

SETS AND REPS

BEGINNER: 1 to 2 sets,
8 to 12 repetitions,
5- to 8-pound dumbbell
INTERMEDIATE: 2 to 3 sets,
8 to 12 repetitions,
8- to 12-pound dumbbell
ADVANCED: 3 sets, 8 to 12 repetitions,
12- to 20-pound dumbbell

STARTING POSITION

Sit on a sturdy chair or bench with your feet flat on the floor. Hold a dumbbell vertically in front of you with both hands, cupping the upper end with your palms facing forward and pinkies up. Sit tall and draw your shoulders back and down. Contract your abdominal muscles. Extend your arms above your head so that the dumbbell is positioned vertically behind your head.

THE MOVE

Bend your elbows and lower the weight behind your head. Flex your wrists at the bottom of the move so you don't hit the back of your neck with the dumbbell. Using your triceps, raise the dumbbell over your head toward the ceiling to complete 1 repetition. Repeat until you complete 1 set.

FOCUS ON FORM

❖ Keep your shoulders down and away from your ears.

❖ Gaze directly in front of you, with your head level and your neck straight.

❖ Keep your wrists close together so that your elbows do not flare out to the sides.

AT HOME/AT THE GYM

AT HOME: If you want more support for your lower back, sit on a chair with back support, like a chair from your kitchen table set. Make sure that you can still lower the dumbbell completely without hitting the chair's back.

AT THE GYM: Try this move while sitting on a stability ball. Contract your abdominals tightly to help you keep your balance.

BEGINNER

Perform the move with one arm at a time, using a lighter dumbbell. Also, brace your working arm by holding it just below the elbow with your other hand.

INTERMEDIATE

Try performing the move with one arm at a time without support. Hold the dumbbell vertically by its bar, with the pinkie side of your hand resting against the top weight's inner plate. Leave your other arm at your side. Repeat until you complete 1 set, then switch arms.

ADVANCED

Add a front shoulder press. Perform the move as described. After the dumbbell is over your head, bring it back in front of your face. Bend your elbows and slowly lower it until it is in front of your chest. Press the dumbbell back up over your head and repeat until you complete 1 set.

ORIGINAL MOVE

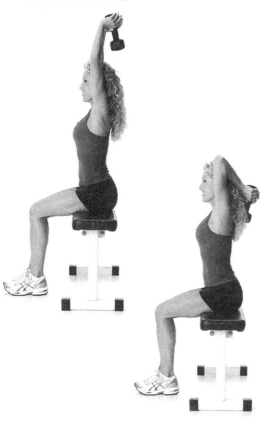

ADVANCED MOVE

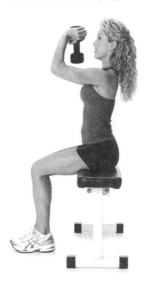

Minna Says

When was the last time you did something for the first time? Never lose the childlike thrill of discovery.

USE YOUR HEAD

If you feel like your shoulders are working harder than your triceps, focus on form. Lift and lower the dumbbell slowly and carefully—really try to isolate those triceps muscles.

Imagine your arms are rubber bands. As you extend them, your wrists are pulled one way and your shoulders the opposite way (down). This keeps your shoulders from working harder than your triceps.

BREATHWORK

Exhale as you lower the dumbbell. Inhale as you lift it over your head.

SUGGESTED STRETCH

Moving Flexibility: Bent-Arm Overhead (page 38)

TRICEPS DIP

This move will improve your arms' "rear view"
by strengthening and toning the triceps.

SETS AND REPS

BEGINNER: 1 to 2 sets,
8 to 12 repetitions
INTERMEDIATE: 2 to 3 sets,
8 to 12 repetitions
ADVANCED: 3 sets, 8 to 12 repetitions

STARTING POSITION

Sit on a sturdy chair or bench. Place your hands, palms down, on the seat on both sides of your bottom, with your fingers pointing forward. Align your hips and shoulders, contract your abdominal muscles, and draw your shoulders back and down. Lift your pelvis off the chair and walk your feet forward to the position indicated for your fitness level.

THE MOVE

Bend your elbows and lower your body until your upper arms are parallel or almost parallel with the floor. Use your triceps to return to the starting position, straightening your arms but not locking your elbows.

FOCUS ON FORM

♣ Lift your chest.
♣ To keep your torso long and tall, draw your shoulders back and down and squeeze the muscles between your shoulder blades.
♣ Keep your backside close to the seat of the chair.

AT HOME/AT THE GYM

AT HOME: If you don't have a sturdy chair or bench, use the bottom stair of a staircase.

AT THE GYM: Use the assisted dip machine. Ask a trainer for assistance if necessary. Or perform this move with a medicine ball. While sitting on the floor, place the ball against your lower back. Reach back and place your hands on the ball. Bend your knees and lift yourself until your bottom is just above the floor. Using your triceps, lift your butt as you straighten your arms. Bend your elbows and lower yourself down again, stopping just before your butt touches the floor. This variation is not for beginners.

BEGINNER

To reduce the amount of body weight you must lift, bend your knees to 90 degrees, positioning your feet directly beneath your knees.

INTERMEDIATE

Perform the move with your knees slightly bent and one foot on top of the other.

ADVANCED

Perform alternating knee bends: Assume the starting position, with your legs extended and straight. As you lower into the dip, bend your left knee and raise it toward your chest. As you return to the starting position, place your left foot on the floor again. Switch legs for the next repetition.

ORIGINAL MOVE

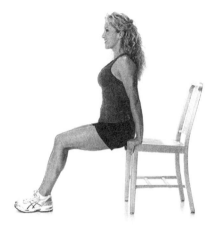

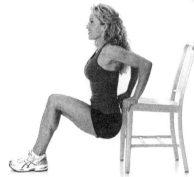

ADVANCED MOVE

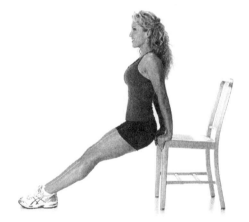

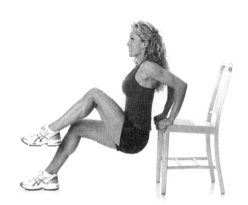

USE YOUR HEAD

The three heads of the triceps muscle—long, lateral, and medial—work together to extend the elbow and straighten the arm. As you perform this move, imagine all three parts working as smoothly as a well-oiled machine to lift and lower your body.

BREATHWORK

Inhale as you lower your body toward the floor. Exhale as you return to the starting position.

ROTATIONAL SHOULDER PRESS

This move rewards you with shapely shoulders—every season's must-have accessory. It sculpts the shoulders, strengthens the biceps, and tones the core.

SETS AND REPS

BEGINNER: 1 to 2 sets,
16 to 24 alternating repetitions,
1- to 5-pound dumbbells
INTERMEDIATE: 2 to 3 sets,
16 to 24 alternating repetitions,
5- to 8-pound dumbbells
ADVANCED: 3 sets,
16 to 24 alternating repetitions,
8- to 12-pound dumbbells

STARTING POSITION

Stand with your feet 2 to 3 feet apart and your knees slightly bent. With your arms at your sides, hold a dumbbell in each hand, palms facing inward. Contract your abdominal muscles, align your hips with your shoulders, and draw your shoulders back and down. Bend your elbows to lift the dumbbells in front of you as shown, palms facing each other.

THE MOVE

Press the dumbbell in your right hand diagonally over your head, toward the left side of your body. Lower your arm to the starting position. Repeat the move with the dumbbell in your left hand. Repeat, alternating repetitions, until you complete 1 set.

FOCUS ON FORM

* Keep your back straight—avoid arching or rounding it.
* Contract your abs throughout the move to support your lower back.
* Keep your shoulders down and away from your ears.

AT HOME/AT THE GYM

AT HOME: Perform this movement without the dumbbells, instead throwing real uppercuts as fast as you can with good form.

AT THE GYM: If your gym has one, try this move on a functional trainer, a cable-based machine that can be adjusted to different planes and heights. Ask a trainer to help you adjust one of the machine's arms to your shoulder height.

BEGINNER

If you wish, sit on a sturdy chair to perform this move, especially if you have back problems.

INTERMEDIATE

Involve your lower body. As you begin to press your right arm upward, squeeze your right glute, lift your right heel off the floor, and pivot your right foot inward to turn your body. Lower the weight, rotate back to the starting position, and switch sides.

ADVANCED

Add a squat to the intermediate move. Bend your knees and lower into a squat, then drive your body upward and rotate to one side as you press the weight up over your head. Return to the squat, then switch sides.

ORIGINAL MOVE

ADVANCED MOVE

Minna Says
Instead of talking yourself out of a workout, talk yourself into one. "You can do it, I *know* you can!"

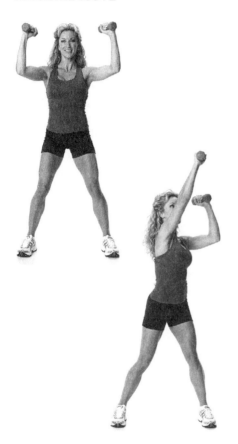

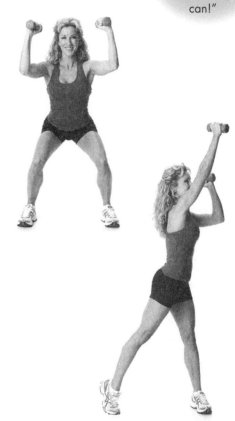

USE YOUR HEAD

This move is slower and more controlled than an uppercut, but imagine the power a boxer releases in each upward punch. Aim for this explosiveness without the speed—as you press upward, contract the muscles in your arms and shoulders as hard as you can.

BREATHWORK

Exhale as you press the dumbbell over your head. Inhale as you lower it to the starting position.

SUGGESTED STRETCH
Static:
Single-Arm Reach Across
(page 26)

✤

CONCENTRATION CURL

This move gives you the right to bare arms.
It shapes and defines the biceps.

SETS AND REPS

BEGINNER: 1 to 2 sets, 8 to 12 repetitions,
3- to 8-pound dumbbell
INTERMEDIATE: 2 to 3 sets,
8 to 12 repetitions,
5- to 10-pound dumbbell
ADVANCED: 3 sets, 8 to 12 repetitions,
8- to 15-pound dumbbell

STARTING POSITION

Sit on a chair or bench, legs apart, holding
a dumbbell in your left hand. Contract
your abdominal muscles and draw your
shoulders back and down. Place your right
hand on your upper right thigh and lean
forward. Lower your left arm between
your legs so that your left triceps (the
back of your upper arm) touches your left
inner thigh and your left palm faces your
right leg.

THE MOVE

Bending your left elbow, lift the dumbbell
toward your left shoulder. Slowly lower
the dumbbell to the starting position.
Repeat to complete 8 to 12 repetitions.
Switch arms and repeat until you complete
1 set.

Minna Says
We don't make
mistakes; we learn
lessons. In life, the
greatest mistake to live
in constant fear of
making one.

FOCUS ON FORM

✤ Be sure to lean forward—that is a
  critical aspect of this move.
✤ To isolate your biceps effectively, make
  sure your triceps—not just your
  elbow—is against your thigh.
✤ Move only your forearm. If your body
  moves, you are lifting too much weight.

AT HOME/AT THE GYM

AT HOME: Perform the move as described
above. If you're an intermediate or advanced reader and you own a stability
ball, try the move while sitting on it.
AT THE GYM: To challenge and improve
your balance, try this move while sitting
on a stability ball. This variation is not for
beginners.

BEGINNER

To ensure that you are contracting your
biceps, place the fingertips of your free
hand on the biceps you are working. If
you are squeezing hard, you will feel it
inflate more than it would if you were
merely curling the dumbbell.

INTERMEDIATE

Stand with your feet shoulder-width apart.
Lower yourself into a squat and let your
left arm hang free between your legs. Perform the move with your arm hanging
free rather than touching your inner knee.
Perform 8 to 12 repetitions, then switch
arms and repeat until you complete 1 set.

ADVANCED

Perform this move while in an advanced Curtsy Lunge stance (see page 187) to engage the muscles of your thighs and your glutes and to challenge your balance. Holding a dumbbell in your right hand, assume the starting position for the advanced Curtsy Lunge stance—right leg forward, left leg back. Place your right triceps against your right inner thigh. Holding the stance, perform the recommended number of concentration curls. Switch sides and repeat until you complete 1 set.

ORIGINAL MOVE

ADVANCED MOVE

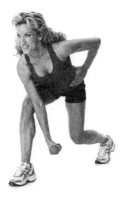

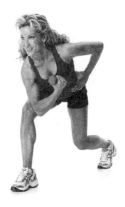

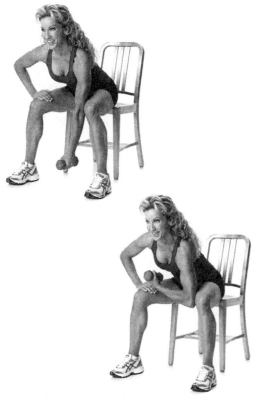

USE YOUR HEAD

As you perform each repetition, visualize your biceps inflating like a balloon. Note its fullness as you contract it during the upward motion. Try to hold on to the fullness as you return to the starting position.

BREATHWORK

Exhale as you curl the dumbbell toward your shoulder. Inhale as you return it to the starting position.

SUGGESTED STRETCH
Moving Flexibility:
Single-Arm Reach Back
(page 39)

CHEST FLY

Few moves define and shape the chest and the fronts of the shoulders—as crucial to tank top appeal as toned arms—like this one.

SETS AND REPS

BEGINNER: 1 to 2 sets, 8 to 12 repetitions, 3- to 5-pound dumbbells

INTERMEDIATE: 2 to 3 sets, 8 to 12 repetitions, 5- to 8-pound dumbbells

ADVANCED: 3 sets, 8 to 12 repetitions, 8- to 15-pound dumbbells

STARTING POSITION

Sit on the floor or on the edge of a bench. Grasp a dumbbell in each hand and rest them on your thighs. Get settled, then lie back with your knees bent and your feet flat on the floor or bench. Contract your abdominal muscles and draw your shoulders down and back. Lift the dumbbells over your head, with your elbows slightly bent and your palms facing each other.

THE MOVE

Keeping your elbows slightly bent, slowly lower your arms toward the floor until the dumbbells are at the level of your shoulders. Hold for a second. Squeeze your chest muscles to return to the starting position and complete 1 repetition.

FOCUS ON FORM

✤ Perform the move in a slow, controlled manner so you do not overstretch your chest or shoulder muscles.

✤ Lower the dumbbells only until they are aligned with your shoulders. Dipping farther won't work your chest muscles any harder and may cause shoulder injury.

✤ Contract the abdominals throughout the move to support your lower back.

AT HOME/AT THE GYM

AT HOME: Try a wall plyometric pushup. Stand facing a wall, 3 to 4 feet away from it, with your feet either hip- or shoulder-width apart. (The closer together your feet, the more challenging the move.) Place your hands on the wall with your arms straight and your wrists aligned with your shoulders. Bending your elbows, lower yourself toward the wall, as if you were performing a pushup. When your elbows are fully bent, push off in an explosive manner so that your hands leave the wall, then allow yourself to return to the wall, bending your elbows as you land.

AT THE GYM: Beginners, try this move on the seated fly machine. Have a trainer help you adjust the machine. Hold the bars with your arms extended to both sides at shoulder height. As you exhale, use your chest and shoulder muscles to bring the bars together so that they almost meet. Inhale and return to the starting position. Intermediate and advanced readers, use the cable crossover machine. Attach the handlebars to the upper pulleys and select the desired weight. Stand with one foot in front of the other. Contract your abdominal muscles. Hold the bars so that your arms extend to both sides at shoulder height. Use your chest and shoulder muscles to pull your hands together; resist the weight as you open your arms again.

BEGINNER

If this move overtaxes your chest and shoulders, replace 1 set of Chest Flys with 1 set of Chest Presses (see page 66).

INTERMEDIATE

Alternate arms to challenge your stability and engage your core. As you lower your right arm, leave your left arm above your head. Return your right arm to the starting position and lower your left arm, leaving your right arm above your head. Repeat, alternating arms, until you complete 1 set.

ADVANCED

Perform the Intermediate move, but challenge your core muscles. Bend your knees to 90 degrees and lift your feet off the floor. Your lower legs should be parallel with the floor and your knees should be directly over your hips.

Minna Says
Fitness isn't a destination. It's a journey. Enjoy the trip.

ORIGINAL MOVE

ADVANCED MOVE

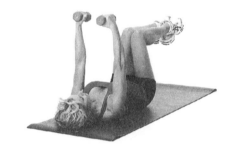

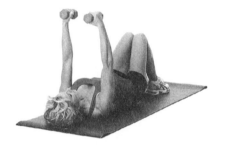

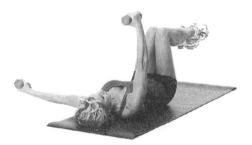

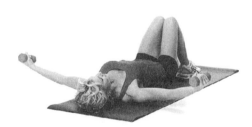

USE YOUR HEAD
Focus on maintaining correct elbow form. They should be neither locked nor bent but slightly cupped, as if you are reaching out for a hug.

BREATHWORK
Inhale as you lower the dumbbells. Exhale as you return to the starting position.

SUGGESTED STRETCH
Moving Flexibility:
Open Arm
(page 41)

3

TANK TOP ARMS
MASTER

If you've graduated from the Skilled moves or have lifted weights for at least a year and want to step up your training, you're ready for these mega-challenging moves. Fortunately, you'll have fun working your upper body to the max. These exercises combine yoga, ballet, sports-style training, and Middle Eastern dance. (I dare you to get bored!) Bonus: Many of these moves work your entire body. The more parts worked, the more calories burned.

  If you are working out at home, you will need a set of dumbbells heavier than those used to perform the Skilled moves, as well as a towel. *Optional:* a Bosu ball or a medicine ball, if you want to perform the variations in the "At the Gym" sections.

FEATURED EXERCISES:
♣PLANK HOLD WALKOUT
♣YOGI PUSHUP
♣ONE-ARM TRICEPS PUSHUP
♣FRONT TO SIDE PLANK
♣BENT-OVER ROW
♣SIDE PLANK WITH ARM RAISE
♣ARNOLD PRESS
♣SHOULDER SHIMMY

PLANK HOLD WALKOUT

This move, which is not your usual shoulder exercise, is one of my best-kept secrets! It strengthens your core, chest, and shoulders and improves shoulder joint integrity.

SETS AND REPS

BEGINNER: 1 to 2 sets,
5 to 10 repetitions per side
INTERMEDIATE: 2 to 3 sets,
5 to 12 repetitions per side
ADVANCED: 3 sets,
8 to 12 repetitions per side

STARTING POSITION

Get down on all fours, with your wrists directly beneath your shoulders and your fingers pointing forward. Extend your legs straight back so that you are at the top of a pushup position (called the Front Plank in yoga). Contract your abdominal muscles; square your shoulders and hips. Maintain one long, straight line from your head to your heels.

THE MOVE

While in the Front Plank position, walk your right hand 6 to 12 inches to the right of your body. Repeat with your left hand, walking it to the left. Walk your right hand back to its starting position beneath your right shoulder, and then walk your left hand back beneath your left shoulder. Repeat, leading with the right hand first (for your prescribed number of reps) and then leading with the left hand to complete 1 set.

Minna Says
Dreaming of the beautiful body you hope to achieve won't get you far. Start by appreciating the beautiful body you have *today.*

FOCUS ON FORM

❧ Contract your abdominal muscles throughout the move.
❧ Keep your shoulders down and away from your ears.
❧ Breathe deeply to help you complete the move. Deep breathing delivers much-needed oxygen to working muscles.

AT HOME/AT THE GYM

AT HOME: Perform the movement as described above. If you're an advanced reader and you own a step bench, perform the move below.

AT THE GYM: Place your left hand on the edge of a step bench positioned in front of you and your right hand on the floor. Perform a pushup. As you straighten your arms, walk your right hand forward onto the bench and your left hand onto the floor. Perform a pushup, then repeat the move, walking your left hand onto the bench and your right hand onto the floor. Repeat, alternating sides. This variation is not for beginners.

BEGINNERS

If you cannot walk your hands while holding the full Front Plank position, kneel instead.

INTERMEDIATE

If you find the full Front Plank position too challenging and the kneeling version not hard enough, assume the full position but keep your feet 2 to 3 feet apart.

ORIGINAL MOVE

ADVANCED

For a major challenge, straighten and lift one leg as you hold the position and perform the move. When leading with your right hand, lift your left leg, and vice versa.

ADVANCED MOVE

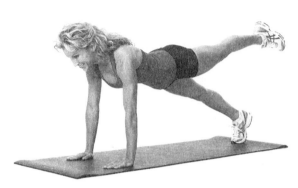

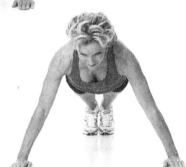

USE YOUR HEAD

Contract every muscle in your body to the hardness of a rock. Speaking of rocks, think about how you might move a very heavy boulder. You would rock it from side to side (likewise, just your body should rock as you walk out your hands), but the rock itself—your body—would not change form, just as your back should not sag or round as you perform this movement.

BREATHWORK

Exhale as you walk your hand out to the side. Inhale as you walk it back in.

SUGGESTED STRETCH
Static:
Single-Arm Reach Across
(page 26)
Moving Flexibility:
Open Arm
(page 41)

YOGI PUSHUP

This move, which requires you to lift your own weight, transforms your body into one extra-large dumbbell. It sculpts the triceps and strengthens the muscles of the chest, shoulders, and core.

SETS AND REPS

BEGINNER: 1 to 2 sets, 8 to 12 repetitions, modified position (see below)
INTERMEDIATE: 2 to 3 sets, 8 to 12 repetitions, wide stance (see below)
ADVANCED: 3 sets, 8 to 12 repetitions, full position

STARTING POSITION

Get down on all fours. Keep your neck and head in a straight line with your back, and look at the floor. Place your wrists directly beneath your shoulders, fingers pointing forward. Extend your legs straight back, with your feet together and only your toes on the floor. Contract your abdominal muscles.

THE MOVE

Keeping your elbows close to your sides, bend your elbows and lower your body until it is 2 to 3 inches from the floor. Using your triceps, press back up to the starting position to complete 1 repetition.

FOCUS ON FORM

✤ Contract your abdominals throughout the move to help your back stay straight.
✤ Distribute your body weight evenly between both hands. Keep most of your weight on the inside of your hands, toward the index finger and thumb, rather than on the outside (toward the pinkie).
✤ If the full position makes your wrists hurt, perform the modified position (see Beginner, below) until your triceps gain strength.

BEGINNER

Try a beginner-friendly version of the full pushup: Instead of balancing on your toes, support yourself on your knees, which should be hip-width apart. Keep your spine aligned so that there is a straight line from your head to your knees.

INTERMEDIATE

Perform the move with your feet 2 to 4 feet apart, rather than together.

ADVANCED

Perform the move on only one leg. Lift the other leg and keep it straight. Halfway through the set, switch legs.

Minna Says

Think only pumping iron strengthens and sculpts muscles? Think again. Moves that use only your body's weight for resistance, such as pushups and situps, also get the job done.

ORIGINAL MOVE

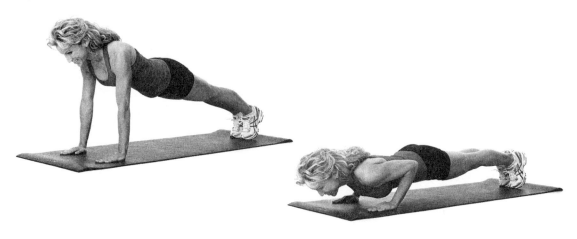

ADVANCED MOVE

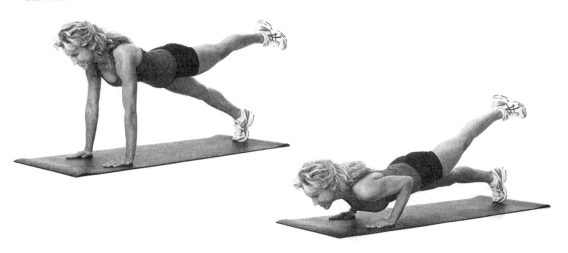

USE YOUR HEAD
To help you isolate the muscles of your triceps, imagine pushing your hands and arms straight through the floor.

BREATHWORK
Inhale as you lower yourself. Exhale as you push up to the starting position.

SUGGESTED STRETCH
Moving Flexibility:
Bent-Arm Overhead
(page 38)

ONE-ARM TRICEPS PUSHUP

This is a killer move, but come on, you can do it! It sculpts the triceps, strengthens the abs and shoulders, and improves balance.

SETS AND REPS

BEGINNER: 1 to 2 sets, 8 to 12 repetitions each side
INTERMEDIATE: 2 to 3 sets, 8 to 12 repetitions each side
ADVANCED: 3 sets, 8 to 12 repetitions each side

STARTING POSITION

Lie on your right side on the floor. Bend your knees slightly and stack your hips and shoulders. Place your right hand on your left hip and your left hand on the floor in front of your right shoulder. Contract your abdominal muscles.

THE MOVE

Pressing your left hand into the floor, straighten your left arm to lift your torso off the floor. You should feel this effort in your triceps. Bend your left elbow to lower your torso toward the floor, but don't let your right shoulder touch the floor. Repeat to finish the prescribed number of reps. Switch sides and repeat to complete one set.

FOCUS ON FORM

✤ Keep your shoulders and hips squared and facing forward.
✤ As you straighten your arm, avoid locking your elbow—keep it soft.
✤ Contract your abdominals throughout the move.

AT HOME/AT THE GYM

AT HOME: Perform a one-arm wall pushup: Stand 3 to 4 feet away from and facing a wall with your feet hip-width apart (hardest) or shoulder-width apart (easier). Place your right hand on the wall. Bending your right elbow, lower yourself toward the wall without bending at the waist or knees. Then push yourself back to the starting position.

AT THE GYM: Try this alternative move on the upper pulley of the cable crossover machine. Attach a handlebar to the upper pulley. Adjust the weight to the desired amount. Stand with your feet hip-width apart, your knees bent, and your abdominals contracted. Grasp the handlebar with your right hand; tuck your right elbow into your side and keep your right wrist straight. Using your triceps, straighten your right arm and press the weight down. Bend your right elbow and resist the weight as you bring your arm back to the starting position. Perform 1 set, then switch arms. If you're performing an odd number of sets, switch arms halfway through each set.

Minna Says
Always believe in yourself—never give up. Your persistence is a measure of your faith in yourself.

BEGINNER

Focus on form: Perform as many repetitions as you can using the correct form.

INTERMEDIATE

Hold your position for 10 to 30 seconds at the bottom of the last repetition in a set before returning to the starting position. Breathe deeply.

ADVANCED

Perform a one-arm full- or wide-stance pushup: Get down on all fours with your hands beneath your shoulders. Extend your legs, positioning your feet hip-width apart or wider on the floor. Your body should be one long, straight line from your head to your heels. Place your right hand halfway between its starting position and your left hand. Lift your left hand off the floor and place it on your lower back. Bend your right elbow and lower your body until it is a few inches from the floor. Using your triceps, push your body back up to the starting position.

ORIGINAL MOVE

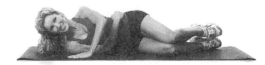

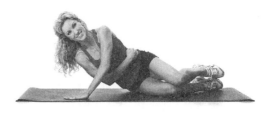

ADVANCED MOVE

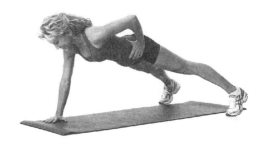

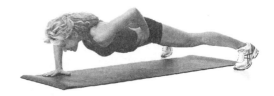

USE YOUR HEAD

Positive reinforcement works with plants, children, and muscles! With each repetition, repeat a positive, present-tense affirmation such as "My triceps are firm, toned, and defined."

BREATHWORK

Exhale as you push upward. Inhale as you lower yourself.

SUGGESTED STRETCH

Moving Flexibility: Bent-Arm Overhead (page 38)

FRONT TO SIDE PLANK

This total body move blasts the obliques, the muscles that run along the sides of your waist. It also strengthens and sculpts the shoulders and strengthens and tones the abdominal and lower back muscles.

SETS AND REPS

BEGINNER: 1 to 2 sets, 16 to 24 alternating repetitions, Front Plank to side lean (see below) INTERMEDIATE: 2 to 3 sets, 16 to 24 alternating repetitions, Front Plank to modified Side Plank in bent-knee position (see opposite page) ADVANCED: 3 sets, 16 to 24 alternating repetitions, Front to Side Plank (see opposite page)

STARTING POSITION

Get down on all fours and assume the Front Plank position (see page 90): Place your palms flat on the floor with your wrists beneath your shoulders, as if you were about to perform a pushup. Extend your legs so that you are balanced on your toes and your body is one long, straight line. Beginners, if necessary, you may start with your knees bent and on the floor, maintaining one long, straight line from your head to your knees.

THE MOVE

Keeping your abdominal muscles tight and your legs straight, lean slightly to the right and begin to rotate your left side upward. BEGINNER: Move into the side lean (see below). INTERMEDIATE: Move into the modified Side Plank in the bent-knee position (see opposite). ADVANCED: Move into the Side Plank (see opposite).

Hold your position for 1 to 3 seconds, then rotate your body back to the Front Plank position. Repeat, leaning to the left and rotating your right side upward. Continue to alternate sides until you complete 1 set.

FOCUS ON FORM

* Keep your body in a straight line by contracting your abdominal, lower back, and gluteal muscles.
* In the Front Plank, distribute your weight evenly between both hands.
* In the Front Plank, keep your shoulders down and away from your ears.
* In the Side Plank, lift your rib cage and contract your abdominal muscles.

AT HOME/AT THE GYM

AT HOME: Perform the move as described above. If you're an advanced reader and you own a stability ball, try the move below.
AT THE GYM: Try the Beginner move with your feet on a stability ball. This variation is not for beginners.

BEGINNER

Follow the Front Plank with the side lean: From the starting position, lean your right shoulder a few inches to the right, either keeping your left hand on the floor or lifting it 1 to 2 inches. Return to the starting position and repeat the move with your left shoulder. Continue, alternating sides, until you complete 1 set.

INTERMEDIATE

As you move into the Side Plank position, drop your right knee to the floor, extend your left leg up and out, and raise your left arm toward the ceiling. Switch sides. Continue, alternating sides, until you complete 1 set.

ADVANCED

In the Front Plank position, bend your elbows and lower yourself down into a pushup as far as you can while maintaining good form. Use your chest, shoulder, and triceps muscles to push

yourself back up and into the Side Plank, raising your left arm toward the ceiling. Continue, alternating sides, until you complete 1 set.

INTERMEDIATE MOVE

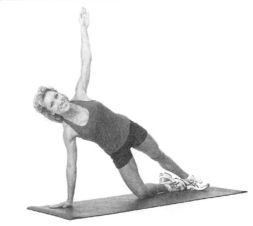

ORIGINAL MOVE

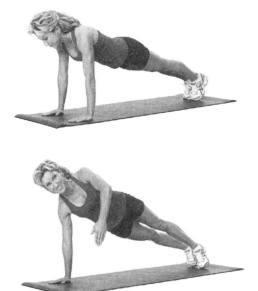

ADVANCED MOVE

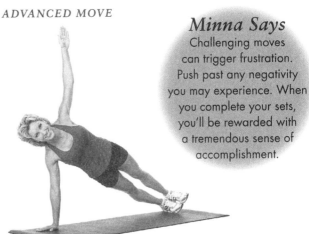

Minna Says

Challenging moves can trigger frustration. Push past any negativity you may experience. When you complete your sets, you'll be rewarded with a tremendous sense of accomplishment.

USE YOUR HEAD

In the Side Plank, extend and lengthen your arm through the fingertips of your raised hand. Imagine that you are reaching for the ceiling with that hand and pushing through the floor with the other.

BREATHWORK

Because this is a challenging move, you may find yourself holding your breath. Throughout the move, focus on breathing deeply and continuously through your nose.

SUGGESTED STRETCH

Static:
Single-Arm Reach Across
(page 26)
Moving Flexibility:
Open Arm
(page 41)

BENT-OVER ROW

This move sculpts a lovely, shapely back for backless dresses and halter tops. It strengthens the back and biceps muscles.

SETS AND REPS

BEGINNER: 1 to 2 sets, 8 to 12 repetitions per side, 5- to 8-pound dumbbell
INTERMEDIATE: 2 to 3 sets, 8 to 12 repetitions per side, 8- to 12-pound dumbbell
ADVANCED: 3 sets, 8 to 12 repetitions per side, 3- to 8-pound dumbbell for the movement described on page 99

STARTING POSITION

Holding a dumbbell in your right hand, stand with your left leg about 3 feet in front of the right and your knees slightly bent. Contract your abdominal muscles, draw your shoulders back and down, and tilt your upper body forward. Place your left hand on your left thigh for back support. Let your right arm hang down, palm facing inward.

THE MOVE

Using your back muscles, bend your right elbow and pull the weight upward and backward, toward your hip. Squeeze your rhomboids (the muscles that pull your shoulder blades together), then slowly return to the starting position.

FOCUS ON FORM

✤ Contract your abdominal muscles throughout the move.
✤ Keep your shoulders down and away from your ears.
✤ As you return to the starting position, continue to squeeze your rhomboids.

AT HOME/AT THE GYM

AT HOME: Try reversing your grip. Instead of positioning your palm inward, turn your hand so that it points forward.
AT THE GYM: Try the seated row. Ask a trainer to help you adjust the rowing machine to your height. Select the desired weight. Place both hands on the handles. At first, keep your arms straight and practice pulling back and pressing down your shoulders, squeezing your rhomboids, without pulling on the handles. Perform 1 set of 10 to 15 of these retractions before performing 1 set of rows.

BEGINNER

If you wish, you can use a chair or bench for support. Stand with your feet hip-width apart, holding the dumbbell in your right hand. Lean forward and place your left hand on the seat. Bend both knees slightly. Perform the move.

Minna Says
Happiness is the result of productive effort.

INTERMEDIATE

Perform the move as described. Before returning to the starting position, perform a Triceps Kickback (see page 58). Repeat until you complete your repetitions, then switch sides.

ORIGINAL MOVE

ADVANCED

Perform the move in the T Pose or the modified T Pose (see page 200). Hold a dumbbell in your right hand and assume the left leg T Pose. Perform the move. Repeat until you finish your reps and then switch sides to complete 1 set.

ADVANCED MOVE

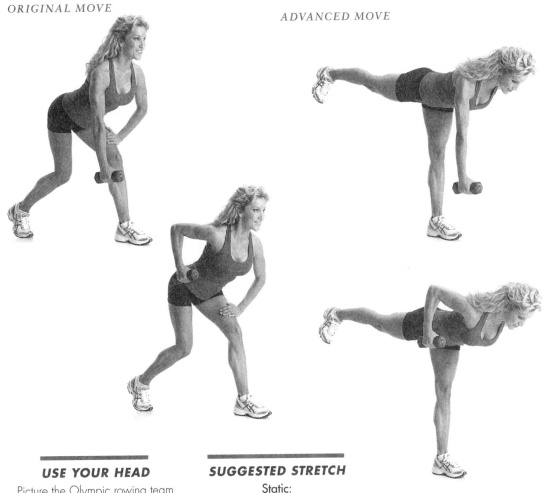

USE YOUR HEAD

Picture the Olympic rowing team performing this move in perfect unison with power and grace.

SUGGESTED STRETCH

Static:
One-Arm Round Front
(page 29)

♣ SIDE PLANK WITH ARM RAISE

This upper body move firms and tightens everything from the shoulders to the back. It defines and tones the shoulders, strengthens the abdominal and lower back muscles, and improves balance and coordination.

SETS AND REPS

BEGINNER: 1 to 2 sets, 8 to 12 repetitions per side, no weight or 3- to 5-pound dumbbell

INTERMEDIATE: 2 to 3 sets, 8 to 12 repetitions per side, 3- to 8-pound dumbbell

ADVANCED: 3 sets, 8 to 12 repetitions per side, 5- to 10-pound dumbbell

STARTING POSITION

Get down on all fours and grasp the dumbbell with your left hand. Extend your legs straight out behind you. Rotate your body so that your left side faces the ceiling as shown.

THE MOVE

While holding the position described above, lift your left arm straight up into the air and over your head, with your palm facing forward. Return to the starting position. Repeat 8 to 12 times, then switch sides to complete 1 set.

FOCUS ON FORM

♣ Contract your abdominal muscles throughout the move to maintain your balance.

♣ Distribute your weight equally between your right foot and your right hand.

♣ Lift through your rib cage and draw your shoulders down and back.

♣ Lift the dumbbell straight up—no zigzagging.

AT HOME/AT THE GYM

AT HOME: Perform the move as described above. If you're advanced and you own a Bosu ball, try the move below.

AT THE GYM: Try this move on the flat side of a Bosu ball with no weight at first, and perhaps never. Position your right hand at the center of the ball. Perform the move. If you can hold the position, raise your left arm. This variation is not for beginners.

BEGINNER

Perform the modified Side Plank: Instead of extending both legs, extend only your left leg and leave your right knee and foot on the floor for balance.

Minna Says
If you think you can't, you won't. If you think you can, you will—and then some.

INTERMEDIATE

Perform the move. Then, as you lower your arm, reach past the starting position toward or past your right hip and twist your torso to engage your abdominal muscles. Return to the starting position. Repeat until you complete the reps, then switch sides to complete 1 set.

ORIGINAL MOVE

ADVANCED

Perform the Intermediate move, but as you raise your arm, lift your left leg as far as you can while keeping your hips and shoulders squared. As you lower your arm, lower your leg and perform the rotation as described. Repeat until you complete the reps, then switch sides to complete 1 set.

ADVANCED MOVE

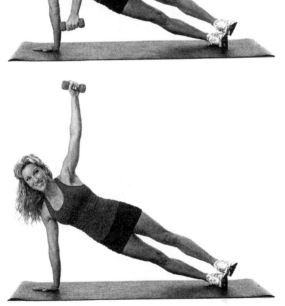

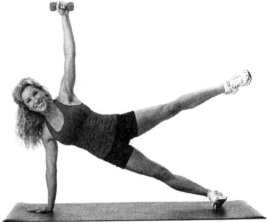

USE YOUR HEAD
Picture yourself as a gymnast who can hold any position without flinching. Only your arm should move as the rest of you stays still, aligned in perfect form.

BREATHWORK
Inhale as you raise your arm. Exhale as you lower it.

SUGGESTED STRETCH
Moving Flexibility:
Child's Pose with Reach Across
(page 42)

ARNOLD PRESS

Even though this move was created by Arnold Schwarzenegger, it won't give you the Terminator's shoulders. Instead, they'll become round and full—very feminine, indeed! This move sculpts and strengthens the deltoid (shoulder) muscles, particularly the anterior deltoid.

SETS AND REPS

BEGINNER: 1 to 2 sets, 8 to 12 repetitions, 3- to 5-pound dumbbells
INTERMEDIATE: 2 to 3 sets, 8 to 12 repetitions, 5- to 10-pound dumbbells
ADVANCED: 3 sets, 8 to 12 repetitions, 8- to 15-pound dumbbells

STARTING POSITION

Sit on a chair or bench, holding the dumbbells on your thighs with your palms facing upward. Contract your abdominal muscles and draw your shoulders back and down. Lift the dumbbells past your shoulders with your palms facing backward.

THE MOVE

Move your still-bent arms out to the sides, away from your body with your elbows pointing to the left and right, and turn the dumbbells so that your palms face forward. As you are doing this, raise the dumbbells over your head. Lower the dumbbells with your arms still out to the sides until your elbows are level with your shoulders. Rotate your still-bent arms to your front, turning the dumbbells so your palms face backwards again to complete 1 repetition. Return to the starting position and repeat until you complete 1 set.

FOCUS ON FORM

- ✤ At the top of the move, keep your elbows soft.
- ✤ As you move your arms to the side, squeeze your shoulder blades together.
- ✤ Keep your shoulders relaxed and away from your ears.
- ✤ Contract your abdominals throughout the move to support your lower back.

AT HOME/AT THE GYM

AT HOME: Perform the move as described above. If you own a stability ball, perform the move below.
AT THE GYM: Perform this move on a stability ball. Sit on the ball, resting the dumbbells on your thighs. Contract your abdominals and draw your shoulders back and down. When you are balanced, lift the dumbbells into the starting position and perform the move.

BEGINNER

If the full move is too intense, perform a basic overhead Shoulder Press. Start with your bent elbows out to the sides at shoulder height to press the dumbbells over your head, keeping your shoulders relaxed and down. Return to the starting position and repeat until you complete 1 set.

Minna Says
Don't strive to fit in when you were born to stand out.

INTERMEDIATE

Try a palms-in variation. Assume the starting position. Instead of moving your arms to the sides and rotating the dumbbells, keep your elbows pointing forward. Press the weights over your head, then lower them until your elbows are at face level, still pointing forward. Using your shoulder muscles, lift your arms straight overhead, then return to the starting position. Repeat until you complete 1 set.

ADVANCED

After performing each set, immediately assume the Modified Plank position (see page 76). Hold it for 10 to 30 seconds.

ORIGINAL MOVE

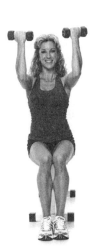 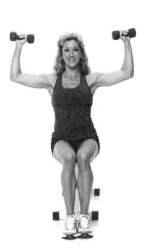 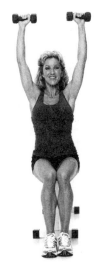

USE YOUR HEAD

I'll be honest: This move can make the front of your shoulders burn like fire. While you should not continue in the face of full-bore pain, you must push past occasional discomfort to achieve peak performance.

BREATHWORK

Exhale as you rotate and press the dumbbells up. Inhale as you lower them.

SUGGESTED STRETCH

Moving Flexibility:
Single-Arm Reach Across
(page 37)
and/or Child's Pose
with Reach Across
(page 42)

♣ SHOULDER SHIMMY

Common in Middle Eastern dance, this move takes great power and stamina.
It also tones the shoulders, strengthens the back, and provides light cardio benefits.

SETS AND REPS

BEGINNER: 2 to 3 sets,
10 to 20 repetitions
INTERMEDIATE: 2 to 3 sets,
10 to 30 repetitions
ADVANCED: 3 sets, work toward
increasing the number of repetitions
and changing the tempo

STARTING POSITION

Stand with your feet together or in a pos-
ing stance (with your weight on your back
leg and the other leg, heel lifted, 12 inches
in front of you). Contract your abdominal
muscles; align your hips and shoulders.
Extend your arms out to your sides to
shoulder height, with your elbows slightly
bent and your palms facing the floor.

THE MOVE

Using your shoulder and chest muscles,
push your right shoulder forward. As you
return your right shoulder to the starting
position, push your left shoulder forward.
Continue this alternating movement until
you complete 1 set.

FOCUS ON FORM

* ♣ Move your shoulders as fully as
  possible and at an even tempo (speed).
* ♣ Push rather than pull each shoulder
  forward.
* ♣ Keep your chest lifted by drawing your
  shoulders back and down.
* ♣ Keep your shoulders relaxed and down
  and away from your ears.

AT HOME/AT THE GYM

AT HOME: To increase this move's cardio
factor, perform it while in the One-Legged
Squat (see page 204) or the Plié Squat (see
page 192).
AT THE GYM: Try this move on a Bosu
ball. Stand on the round side of the ball
with your feet together. Move each
shoulder slowly, using the fullest range of
motion. This variation is for intermediate
and advanced readers only.

BEGINNER

At first this move may place more demands
on your balance and coordination than on
your muscles. Focus on perfecting your
form.

Minna Says
Have the courage to
reach for the stars . . .
and miss. Success
isn't always in the
achievement but in the
effort to achieve.

INTERMEDIATE

Work to increase your shimmying speed. Remember, the idea is to shake your shoulders, not your breasts (which go along for the ride).

ADVANCED

Alternate tempos: Shimmy your shoulders as fast as you can, slow the tempo a bit, then pick up the pace again. Work up to a 60-second shimmy.

ORIGINAL MOVE

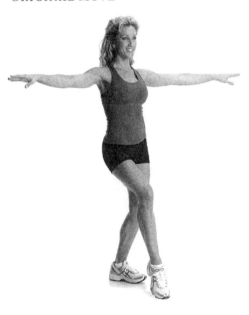

USE YOUR HEAD

Belly dancers make this move look effortless. Picture a dancing girl doing the shimmy—her shoulders vibrate rapidly but in a relaxed manner.

BREATHWORK

Inhale and exhale deeply and continuously throughout the move.

SUGGESTED STRETCH

Static:
Single-Arm Reach Across
(page 26)
Moving Flexibility:
Open Arm (page 41)

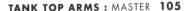

PART 2

BIKINI *Belly*

There's more to getting a bikini belly than performing crunches. You have to work your entire core, which includes the muscles of your abdomen, back, hips, and pelvis.

Every move originates from your core. So many muscles comprise it—29, to be exact—that I won't name them all. A few of the most important, however, are the rectus abdominis, or "six-pack"; the obliques, the muscles that run along the sides of your waist; and the transverse abdominis, the deepest muscle layer in the abdominal wall. Contracting the transverse abdominis compresses the abdomen, and strengthening it helps your stomach to lay nice and flat.

If you're looking to whittle your waist and lose those love handles, the moves in this section can help whether you're new to exercise or a fitness fanatic. In no time at all, you'll be breaking out the low-riders and bikinis to flaunt your taut, toned belly.

NOVICE	SKILLED	MASTER
BASIC CRUNCH	TOTAL BODY CRUNCH	SCISSORS
DOUBLE LEG LIFT	WALKING PLANK	ORIGAMI CRUNCH
BOAT POSE	DIPPING TOES IN WATER	SIDE PLANK
ROLLING BALL	SUPERMAN	GYMNAST ABS
FUNKY ABS	ROLL-UP	ARM AND LEG EXTENSION
1-2-3 CRUNCH!	ROLL BACK AND REACH	REVERSE PLANK
LYING SIDE BEND	BALLERINA TWIST	KNEE DROP
BASIC OBLIQUE TWIST	BICYCLE	TWIST AND DROP

4

BIKINI BELLY
NOVICE

Think you need to do 500 crunches a day to get fab abs? Think again, beginners. While it is effective, the crunch isn't the only move that can deliver the slim, toned midsection you want. The moves in this chapter will whittle away at a jiggly belly for a noticeable change in 4 weeks or less. (Of course, you'll get the best results if you combine this workout with at least 30 minutes of aerobic exercise on most or all days of the week.)

If you are working out at home, you'll need a Bosu ball and/or a stability ball if you wish to try the variations in the "At the Gym" sections.

FEATURED EXERCISES:

♣BASIC CRUNCH

♣DOUBLE LEG LIFT

♣BOAT POSE

♣ROLLING BALL

♣FUNKY ABS

♣1-2-3 CRUNCH!

♣LYING SIDE BEND

♣BASIC OBLIQUE TWIST

BASIC CRUNCH

This move isn't fancy, but it sculpts killer abs by toning and strengthening them.

SETS AND REPS

BEGINNER: 1 to 2 sets, 10 to 20 repetitions
INTERMEDIATE: 2 to 3 sets, 10 to 20 repetitions
ADVANCED: 3 sets, 10 to 20 repetitions

STARTING POSITION

Lie on your back with your knees bent and your feet flat on the floor. Place your hands behind your head, fingertips touching but not interlaced (interlocking your fingers behind your neck can cause injuries), or cross them on your chest.

THE MOVE

Contract your abdominal muscles, then curl your torso forward until your shoulder blades are off the floor. Slowly return to the starting position, maintaining the tension in your abdominals, to complete 1 repetition.

FOCUS ON FORM

❖ The important thing is not how high you lift but, rather, how hard you contract your abs.
❖ Focus on the quality of the contraction, raising your torso only until your shoulder blades leave the floor.
❖ Keep your shoulders down and away from your ears.
❖ Perform the move in a slow, controlled manner.

AT HOME/AT THE GYM

AT HOME: Contract your abs and draw your navel toward your spine throughout the day—as you work at your desk, watch TV, prepare dinner. This will help you develop strong, defined abs more quickly.
AT THE GYM: Perform the move on a stability ball. Lie faceup on the ball with your head, neck, and shoulders off the ball. Bend your knees to 90 degrees and keep your feet flat on the floor. Place your hands behind your head, fingertips touching but not interlaced, or cross them on your chest. Perform the number of repetitions and sets recommended for your fitness level.

BEGINNER

If your neck gets tired, place a small towel behind it, holding one end in each hand. Perform the move with your head and neck resting comfortably on the towel.

INTERMEDIATE

Assume the starting position, but extend your arms over your head in line with your ears, the back of your left hand resting on your right palm. (If you have the strength, keep your hands apart.) Perform the move.

ADVANCED

Perform the Intermediate move described above. At the "top" of the movement, when you are curled up, try adding 10 to 20 pulses, contracting your muscles rhythmically, before returning to the starting position.

ORIGINAL MOVE

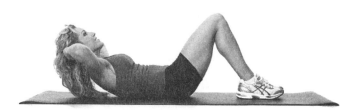

ADVANCED MOVE

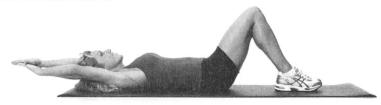

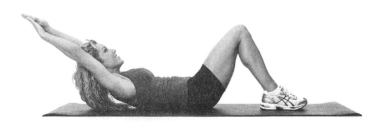

USE YOUR HEAD

Picture your abdominals as an accordion, with your ribs "pleating" toward your hip bone like an accordion's bellows.

BREATHWORK

Exhale as you contract your abdominals and lift your shoulder blades off the floor. Inhale as you slowly return to the starting position.

SUGGESTED STRETCH

Static:

Cobra Pose
(page 32)

DOUBLE LEG LIFT

No need to do hundreds of crunches—this move sculpts sleek, sexy abs in less than 5 minutes by toning the rectus abdominis muscle, or "six-pack."

SETS AND REPS

BEGINNER: 1 to 2 sets, 10 to 15 repetitions with knees bent (see below)
INTERMEDIATE: 2 to 3 sets, 10 to 15 repetitions
ADVANCED: 3 sets, 10 to 15 repetitions

STARTING POSITION

Lie on your back, knees bent, arms at your sides, and palms flat on the floor. Lift your legs straight up over your hips, toes pointing toward the ceiling.

THE MOVE

Contract your abdominal muscles, then use them to lift your pelvis off the floor. Keep your legs pointing straight up in the air. Dropping them forward or leaning them back lessens the effectiveness of this exercise. Slowly return to the starting position, maintaining the tension in your abdominal muscles, to complete 1 repetition.

FOCUS ON FORM

♣ Use only your abdominals to perform the move. Press your palms into the floor to work your triceps.
♣ Avoid pushing out your abs in an attempt to lift your pelvis off the floor. If you can't lift your pelvis without pushing out your abs, simply contract them without raising your pelvis to work your abs instead.

AT HOME/AT THE GYM

AT HOME: Perform the move as described above. If you own a stability ball, try the move below.
AT THE GYM: Hold a stability ball between your legs (the closer the ball is to your feet, the more challenging the move will be for your abdominal muscles). Perform the move as described.

BEGINNER

To make the move easier, try this variation: Instead of lifting your legs straight up, bend your knees and lift your feet off the floor so your knees are aligned over your hips and your feet and lower legs are parallel with the floor. Then raise your pelvis and perform the move.

INTERMEDIATE

Keep your pelvis off the floor throughout each set so you aren't resting between repetitions.

ADVANCED

Perform the Intermediate move as described. As you hold the last repetition at the top of the move, contract your muscles in a pulsing motion 10 to 15 times.

ORIGINAL MOVE

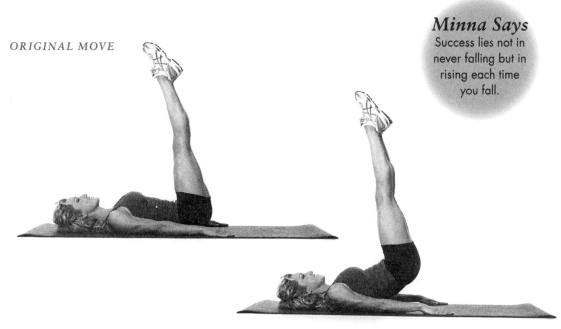

BEGINNER MOVE

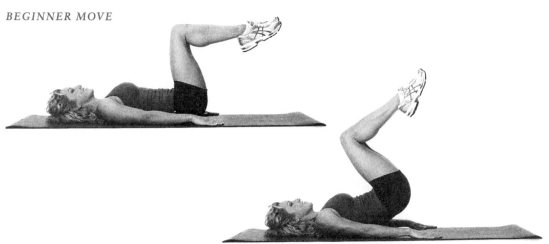

USE YOUR HEAD

Imagine that a rope tied around your ankles is slowly lifting your legs and pelvis off the floor, then slowly lowering them again in exactly the same alignment for every repetition.

BREATHWORK

Exhale as you lift your legs into the air. Inhale as you return to the starting position.

SUGGESTED STRETCH
Moving Flexibility:
Lunge with One-Arm Reach (page 43)

BOAT POSE

This move combines core and balance work—and your abs will feel the heat! It tightens and tones the abdominal muscles and strengthens the hip flexors and quadriceps.

SETS AND REPS

BEGINNER: 1 to 2 sets, hold for 5 to 15 seconds with your feet on the floor (see opposite page)
INTERMEDIATE: 2 to 3 sets, hold for 10 to 20 seconds
ADVANCED: 3 sets, hold for 15 to 30 seconds

STARTING POSITION

Sit tall on your sit bones on the floor with your knees bent and your feet flat on the floor. Contract your abdominals and pull your navel in toward your spine. Align your hips and shoulders and draw your shoulders back and down. Grasp the outer sides of your thighs.

THE MOVE

Keeping your abs tight and your spine long and straight, lean back on your sit bones and lift both feet off the floor. Keep your knees bent and lift until your lower legs are parallel with the floor (you should look like a boat). Hold, breathing deeply, for the amount of time indicated for your fitness level. Repeat until you complete 1 set.

FOCUS ON FORM

❖ Expect to wobble until you gain the core strength to hold this position.
❖ The key is to keep your spine long. Lengthen yourself as much as possible from your head to your tailbone.
❖ Keep your shoulders down and away from your ears.
❖ Contract your abdominals throughout the move.

AT HOME/AT THE GYM

AT HOME: Try a fusion of this move with the Rolling Ball exercise (see page 116). Perform the Rolling Ball as directed. At the top of the move, straighten your back, lift your lower legs until they are parallel with the floor, and hold for a count of three to five. Then tuck your lower legs so that your heels are close to your butt and roll back again. Repeat until you complete 1 set.

AT THE GYM: Attempt this on the Bosu ball. Sit in the center of the ball, round side up, and perform the move. This variation is for advanced exercisers only.

Minna Says
Rome wasn't built in a day, and neither is a tight, toned body. Stop looking in the mirror for a week or two. Progress becomes more apparent when we stop looking so hard for it.

BEGINNER

Keep your feet flat on the floor and practice leaning back with perfect form (long spine, tight abdominals). Focus on keeping your back rail-straight and your abs rock hard as you lean back. When you can do this, graduate to lifting your legs.

INTERMEDIATE

Try to take your hands off your thighs. This will present a serious challenge to your balance, but it'll also turn up the heat on your abs.

ADVANCED

Perform the Intermediate move as described, then extend your legs straight up into the air so that your torso and legs create a tight V shape. Stay long in your spine. If you round your back, you'll lose the abdominal workout.

ORIGINAL MOVE

ADVANCED MOVE

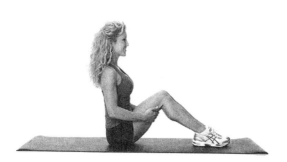

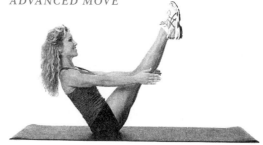

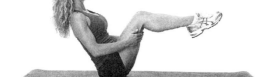

USE YOUR HEAD

Picture yourself as a small boat. After navigating through rough waters (finding your balance, gaining core strength), you'll find calmer seas and float effortlessly, as still as the water is.

BREATHWORK

Breathe deeply in and out through your nose, inhaling so that the air hits the back of your throat.

SUGGESTED STRETCH

Moving Flexibility:
Lunge with One-Arm Reach
(page 43)

ROLLING BALL

This is one of my favorite abdominal moves because it doubles as a back massage.
It also strengthens the abdominals, increases core strength, and improves balance.

SETS AND REPS

BEGINNER: 1 to 2 sets, 8 to 12 repetitions
INTERMEDIATE: 2 to 3 sets,
8 to 12 repetitions
ADVANCED: 3 sets, 8 to 12 repetitions

STARTING POSITION

Sit tall on your sit bones on the floor, legs together, knees drawn in toward your chest, heels near your butt. Wrap your arms around your legs, placing each palm on the shin on the same side and keeping your elbows at your sides. Contract your abdominals, drawing your navel toward your spine, and tuck your pelvis so that you create the letter C from the top of your head to the base of your spine. (This position is called the C-curve.) Lift your feet and lean back so that you are balancing on your spine just above your tailbone.

THE MOVE

Look at your navel, inhale, and roll back, like a ball, onto your shoulder blades. Maintain the C-curve and keep your shoulders, neck, and head off the mat.

Keeping your feet off the floor, exhale as you return to the starting position to complete 1 repetition.

FOCUS ON FORM

* Roll on your upper back only; your head and neck should not touch the floor.
* Maintain the contraction in your abs throughout the move.
* Elongate your neck, relax your shoulders, and imagine moving your ribs toward your hip bones.

AT HOME/AT THE GYM

AT HOME: Try a basic Pilates move called "the hundreds." Lie on your back on the floor with your knees tucked to your chest; lightly grasp your ankles. Contract your abdominals, lift your head and shoulders off the floor, and straighten your arms at your sides, palms down, 6 inches from the floor. Extend and raise your legs to between 45 degrees off the floor (most challenging) and vertical; keeping your heels together and your toes pointed, rotate your thighs outward. Hold as you quickly inhale 5 times and then quickly exhale 5 times. At the same time, bounce your arms in unison with your breathing—palms upward on the inhalations and downward on the exhalations. Repeat 10 times for a total of 100 breaths.
AT THE GYM: Try balancing on a Bosu ball as you perform only the C-curve part of the move.

Minna Says
Goals are like sweet, sun-warmed strawberries— you can't have just one. Set several mini-goals that you can achieve on your way to your ultimate goal.

BEGINNER

Focus first on learning to execute the perfect C-curve. It's this technique that works your abdominals.

INTERMEDIATE

Try keeping your legs and heels farther apart, closer to hip-width.

ADVANCED

Each time you roll up, find your balance point, then hold the Boat Pose (see page 114). Hold for 3 to 5 seconds. This is a demanding move because your body must switch from the rounded spine of the C-curve to the elongated spine of the Boat Pose.

ORIGINAL MOVE

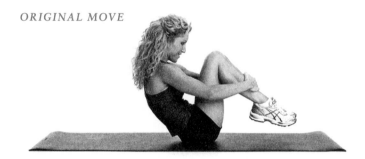

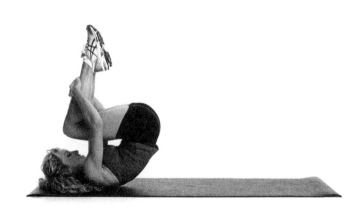

USE YOUR HEAD

Focus on maintaining a strong C-curve. Imagine that a string attached to your navel is pulling it toward your spine.

BREATHWORK

Inhale as you roll back. Exhale as you return to the starting position.

SUGGESTED STRETCH
Static:
Cobra Pose
(page 32)

FUNKY ABS

A staple of hip-hop dance choreography, this move is a fun, funked-up way to tone your abs. It sculpts your abdominal muscles, strengthens your lower back, and improves coordination.

SETS AND REPS

BEGINNER: 1 to 2 sets,
10 to 15 slow repetitions,
or yoga version (see opposite page)
INTERMEDIATE: 2 to 3 sets,
10 to 15 repetitions each of slow and fast movements (see opposite page)
ADVANCED: 3 sets,
each 30 to 60 seconds long

STARTING POSITION

Stand with your feet hip- or shoulder-width apart. Bend your knees slightly, contract your abdominal muscles to draw your navel toward your spine, and keep your shoulders relaxed and down.

THE MOVE

Contract your abs even harder, then tilt your pelvis backward, so that you round your back. Using your back muscles, reverse the motion—tilt your pelvis forward so that you stick out your backside. Repeat the backward-forward movement until you complete 1 set.

FOCUS ON FORM

- ♣ Essentially, this move is about using your abdominal muscles to alternately round and arch your back.
- ♣ Throughout the move, contract your abdominal muscles as hard as you can.
- ♣ Tilt your pelvis within your range of flexibility so that you do not stress your lower back.
- ♣ Keep your shoulders down and away from your ears.

AT HOME/AT THE GYM

AT HOME: Try core circles. Stand with your feet shoulder-width apart. Bend your knees slightly. Place your palms on your thighs with your fingers pointing toward each other. Circle clockwise first—push out your rib cage toward your left hip, then do a half-circle around to your right hip and continue the circle back, really drawing in your abdominals as you half-circle back to your left hip. Perform 1 set of 8 to 12 circles clockwise, then circle counterclockwise for 1 set.

AT THE GYM: Try the Beginner move on the flat side of a Bosu ball. First, position your hands and knees at the edge of the ball and find your balance.

Minna Says
Inspiration comes
from others.
Motivation comes
from within.

BEGINNER

Try the yoga version of this move: Get down on all fours. Contract your abdominals and round your back, like a cat does when stretching, exhaling as you do so. Then arch your back and stretch upward, letting your abdominals relax and stretch.

INTERMEDIATE

Combine 10 to 15 slow and 10 to 15 fast repetitions of the move. Play with the tempo—speed up, slow down—and try to keep the shake going.

ADVANCED

Do the move with your arms over your head. Try to keep your palms together as you move as fast as you can. Or add a step-touch aerobic dance step: As you perform this move, step to the side with your right foot, bring your left foot to meet your right, then step to the left and bring your right foot to meet your left.

ORIGINAL MOVE

ADVANCED MOVE

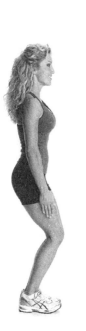
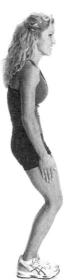
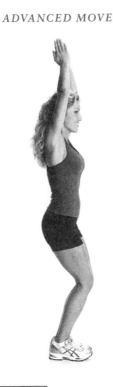
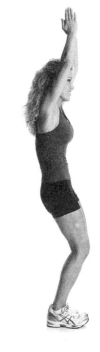

USE YOUR HEAD

The singer Beyoncé is the diva of the derriere shake. Picture yourself as an extra in one of her videos.

BREATHWORK

Inhale and exhale deeply and rhythmically through your nose throughout the move.

SUGGESTED STRETCH

Static:
Child's Pose with Reach Across
(page 30)

1-2-3 CRUNCH!

Toning your abs is as simple as 1-2-3! The contraction phase will challenge your abs until they tremble, but it will reward you with a sleek, sexy six-pack by tightening, toning, and strengthening them.

SETS AND REPS

BEGINNER: 1 to 2 sets, 10 to 15 repetitions

INTERMEDIATE: 2 to 3 sets, 10 to 15 repetitions, arms extended (see opposite page)

ADVANCED: 3 sets, 10 to 15 repetitions, arms and legs fully extended (see opposite page)

STARTING POSITION

Lie on your back with your feet flat on the floor. Place your hands behind your head, with your fingertips touching but not interlaced, or cross them on your chest.

THE MOVE

Contract your abdominals and draw your navel toward your spine. Curl your torso forward over a count of three, until your shoulder blades leave the floor. Return to the starting position, counting backward from three to one, to complete 1 repetition. Be sure to maintain tension in your abdominals throughout the movement.

FOCUS ON FORM

✤ Although you are counting as you lift your torso, lift in a smooth, continuous motion rather than jerking upward as you count.

✤ Contract your abdominals as hard as you can throughout the move. The important thing is not how high you lift but how hard you tighten your abs.

✤ As you lower your torso, maintain the tension in your abdominals. Try to avoid resting your abs (i.e., do not lower yourself completely to the floor) between repetitions.

✤ Keep your shoulders down and away from your ears.

✤ Keep your neck long and avoid tucking your chin into your chest.

AT HOME/AT THE GYM

AT HOME: Try a quicker curl: Lift on a count of one and take a count of three to return to the starting position.

AT THE GYM: Try this move on a stability ball. Lie with your back and shoulders on the ball and your head and neck hanging off it. Perform the move.

BEGINNER

Focus on using proper form. Don't get frustrated if you are unable to lift your torso very high off the floor. If the move proves too challenging, perform the Basic Crunch (see page 110) to complete your sets.

Minna Says
You can wish and always chase your dream, or act and make that dream a reality.

INTERMEDIATE

Perform the move with your arms extended over your head and held close to your ears. Place one palm over the other or—if you have the strength—keep your hands separated.

ADVANCED

Perform the Intermediate move and extend your legs to a position between 45 degrees off the floor and vertical, over your hips. You'll need considerable abdominal strength for this one!

ORIGINAL MOVE

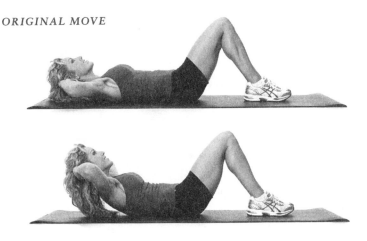

INTERMEDIATE MOVE

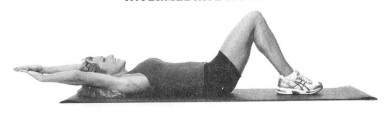

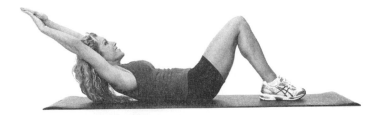

USE YOUR HEAD
Imagine that with each repetition, you are chiseling your six-pack to sculpted perfection.

BREATHWORK
Exhale as you lift your torso on a count of three. Inhale as you lower it.

SUGGESTED STRETCH
Static:
Cobra Pose
(page 32)

LYING SIDE BEND

This move creates a trim, tight waistline you'll want to show off in low-rise jeans. It chisels the abdominal muscles, particularly the rectus abdominis and obliques.

SETS AND REPS

BEGINNER: 1 to 2 sets,
10 to 15 repetitions per side
INTERMEDIATE: 2 to 3 sets,
10 to 15 repetitions per side
ADVANCED: 3 sets,
10 to 15 repetitions per side

STARTING POSITION

Lie on your right side. Stack your hips and shoulders. Place your hands behind your head with your fingertips touching but not interlaced and your elbows pointing forward. Rest your head on your arm.

THE MOVE

Using your abdominals, lift your head and right shoulder as high off the floor as you can. Return to the starting position to complete 1 repetition. Repeat to complete 10 to 15 repetitions, then switch sides to complete 1 set.

FOCUS ON FORM

- ❖ Align your head and spine throughout the move.
- ❖ Keep your shoulders down and away from your ears.
- ❖ Keep your shoulders and hips stacked throughout the move.

AT HOME/AT THE GYM

AT HOME: Perform the Side Plank (see page 150) in the modified position. Lie on the floor on your right side. Raise your hips off the floor and support your weight on your right forearm and right foot, with your elbow directly beneath your shoulder and your forearm perpendicular to your body. Your body should be completely off the floor and form one long, straight line from your head to your heels. From this position, lower your right hip to the floor, then, using your obliques, lift your body again into one long, straight line. Repeat until you complete your reps, then switch sides to complete 1 set.

AT THE GYM: Perform the move on a stability ball with your feet pressed flat against the wall for added support and balance.

BEGINNER

Instead of placing your hands behind your head, place your left palm flat on the floor in front of your chest to help you lift your shoulder off the floor.

INTERMEDIATE

From the starting position, bend your bottom (right) knee but leave your top (left) leg extended. Then perform the move.

ADVANCED

Perform the Intermediate version of this move, but lift your left leg 6 to 12 inches off the floor as you lift your right shoulder.

ORIGINAL MOVE

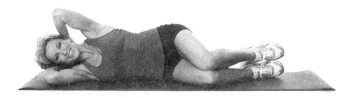

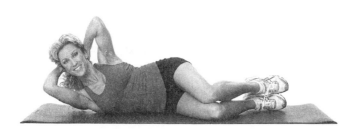

ADVANCED MOVE

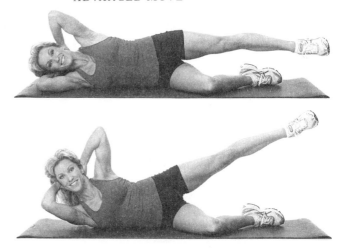

USE YOUR HEAD

As you perform each repetition, imagine that a rope tied around your torso is lifting it up while your hips and legs remain on the floor.

BREATHWORK

Exhale as you lift your shoulder off the floor. Inhale as you lower yourself into the starting position.

SUGGESTED STRETCH

Static:

Spinal Twist
(page 31)

BASIC OBLIQUE TWIST

Twist and turn your way into the teeniest bikini with this fun move. It tones and defines the sides of the abdomen by working the obliques, which allow the torso to twist.

SETS AND REPS

BEGINNER: 1 to 2 sets,
10 to 15 repetitions per side
INTERMEDIATE: 2 to 3 sets,
20 to 30 alternating repetitions
(see opposite page)
ADVANCED: 3 sets, 10 to 15 repetitions
per side with straight-leg lower and lift
(see opposite page)

STARTING POSITION

Lie on your back with your knees bent and
your feet flat on the floor. Place your right
arm by your side with your palm flat on
the floor. Place your left hand behind your
neck, with your left elbow out to the side.
Contract your abdominals by drawing
your navel in toward your spine, then lift
your torso so that your head and shoulders
leave the floor.

THE MOVE

Using your obliques, lift and twist your
torso as far toward your right hip and
knee as you can without tugging on your
head or neck. Return to the starting position to complete 1 repetition. If you are a
beginning or advanced reader, repeat until
you complete your reps, then switch sides
to complete 1 set. If you are
exercising at an intermediate level, alternate sides
with each repetition.

FOCUS ON FORM

✤ Direct your shoulder (rather than your
  elbow) toward the opposite hip or knee.
  Keep your left elbow cocked out to the
  side.
✤ Contract your abdominal muscles hard,
  really drawing your navel toward your
  spine, to tone the deepest muscle layers.
✤ Keep your shoulders down and away
  from your ears.

AT HOME/AT THE GYM

AT HOME: Perform the move as described
above. If you own a stability ball, perform
the move below.
AT THE GYM: Place a stability ball 3 to 4
feet from a wall. Sit on the ball facing the
wall and walk your feet forward until
your back and shoulders are on the ball
and the soles of your feet are braced
against the wall. Place your hands behind
your head. Push the soles of your feet into
the wall to help you balance. Lift and
twist your torso and crunch toward your
right hip. Return to the starting position.
Repeat, then switch sides to complete 1
set. This variation is for intermediate and
advanced readers only.

Minna Says
I love this line from the
movie *Gladiator:* "What
we do today echoes in
eternity." Make your every
word, thought, and deed
foster your success.

BEGINNER

Try to keep your neck and head off the floor throughout the move. Avoid resting your head on the floor between repetitions.

INTERMEDIATE

Try this move with both hands behind your head, and do not rest between repetitions. Alternate sides with each repetition, trying to keep your shoulders, neck, and head off the floor.

ADVANCED

Add a straight-leg lower and lift: From the starting position, extend your right leg straight, keeping your left knee bent and your left foot on the floor. As you lift and twist to the right, lift your right leg, keeping it straightened, to "meet" your left shoulder. Return to the starting position, lowering your right leg as far as you can while still maintaining the contraction in your abdominals. Repeat until you complete your reps, then switch sides to complete 1 set.

ORIGINAL MOVE

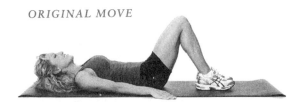

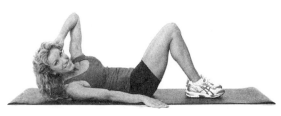

ADVANCED MOVE

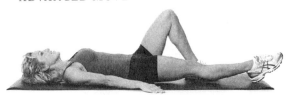

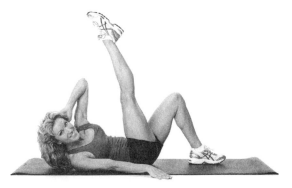

USE YOUR HEAD

Picture a rope connecting your left shoulder to your right knee. As you twist, the rope will loosen like a clothesline being lowered. As you return to the starting position, the rope will become taut.

BREATHWORK

Exhale as you lift and turn your torso. Inhale as you return to the starting position.

SUGGESTED STRETCH

Static:
Cobra Pose (page 32)
Moving Flexibility:
Kneeling Lunge (page 35)

5

BIKINI BELLY
SKILLED

Ready to take your abs to the next level? If you've mastered the Novice Bikini Belly moves, these more challenging abdominal and core exercises are for you. They include a variety of fun styles—Pilates, yoga, ballet—and target your abdominal muscles in ways they may not be used to. The benefit of this element of surprise: faster results. You'll need a mat, plus medicine, Bosu, and stability balls if you want to perform the variations in the "At the Gym" sections.

FEATURED EXERCISES:
♣TOTAL BODY CRUNCH
♣WALKING PLANK
♣DIPPING TOES IN WATER
♣SUPERMAN
♣ROLL-UP
♣ROLL BACK AND REACH
♣BALLERINA TWIST
♣BICYCLE

TOTAL BODY CRUNCH

This total body move totally transforms your abs into a rippling six-pack by strengthening and toning them.

SETS AND REPS

BEGINNER: 1 to 2 sets,
10 to 15 repetitions
INTERMEDIATE: 2 to 3 sets,
10 to 15 repetitions
ADVANCED: 3 sets, 10 to 20 repetitions

STARTING POSITION

Lie on your back on the floor. Lift your legs by bending your knees to 90 degrees and aligning them over your hips. Cock your arms to the sides like wings. Your hands may be either at the sides of your head, with your fingertips on your temples, or behind your neck, with your fingertips touching but not interlaced.

THE MOVE

Using your abdominal muscles, simultaneously lift your shoulders and your pelvis off the floor, bringing your knees toward your shoulders. Slowly return to the starting position to complete 1 repetition.

FOCUS ON FORM

✤ Maintain the contraction in your abdominal muscles throughout the move.
✤ Keep your shoulders down and away from your ears.
✤ Keep your head immobile. Tugging with your hands on the back of your neck to assist your muscles will not work your abs and can strain your neck and spine.
✤ Keep your knees positioned over your hips.

AT HOME/AT THE GYM

AT HOME: Perform the move as described above. Intermediate and advanced readers, if you have someone to help you, try the move below.

AT THE GYM: This move requires an assistant. Try to be an unfoldable folding chair: At the top of the move, bring your elbows inward and touch them to your knees. Have the person assisting you grasp your ankles, *slowly* pull you up into a sitting position, then slowly lower you back down. Keep your elbows glued to your knees throughout and breathe slowly and deeply. This move, which is not for beginners, is a mega-challenge; if you can do even 1 repetition, pat yourself on the back.

BEGINNER

If you cannot lift both your shoulders and your pelvis off the floor, lift your shoulders first, then lift your pelvis. As you return to the starting position, lower your shoulders and pelvis at the same time.

INTERMEDIATE

Try to keep your shoulders slightly off the floor as you return to the starting position so that your abs will remain contracted between repetitions.

ADVANCED

As you return to the starting position, extend and straighten both your arms and your legs. Keep your legs high off the floor and your arms by your ears.

ORIGINAL MOVE

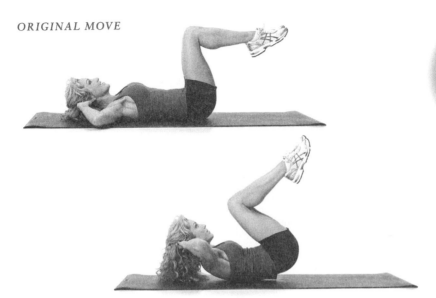

ADVANCED MOVE

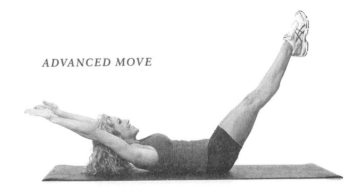

USE YOUR HEAD

When bringing your knees toward your shoulders, picture yourself as a compact ball. The tighter you squeeze your abdominals, the smaller and more compact you become.

BREATHWORK

Exhale as you bring your knees toward your shoulders. Inhale as you return to the starting position.

SUGGESTED STRETCH

Static:
Cobra Pose
(page 32)
Moving Flexibility:
Kneeling Lunge
(page 35)

WALKING PLANK

Adding the walking move to the plank takes your abs to the next level of burn. This move strengthens and tones the core, chest, and shoulder muscles and improves balance and coordination.

SETS AND REPS

BEGINNER: 1 to 2 sets,
5 to 10 repetitions per leading leg
INTERMEDIATE: 2 to 3 sets,
5 to 10 repetitions per leading leg
ADVANCED: 3 sets,
5 to 10 repetitions per leading leg

STARTING POSITION

Get down on all fours. Lower yourself onto your forearms, place your palms flat on the floor, and extend your legs straight back, balancing on your toes. Align your elbows directly beneath your shoulders; angle your hands toward each other and allow your thumbs to touch. Contract your abdominals and square your hips and shoulders. Your body should form one long, straight line from your head to your heels. You are now in the Modified Plank position (see page 76).

THE MOVE

While in the Modified Plank position, walk your left foot out to the side. Repeat with your right foot, so that your feet are a few feet apart. Walk your left foot back to the starting position, then your right. Repeat, leading with your left foot, until you complete 5 to 10 reps, then switch sides, leading with your right foot. Complete 5 to 10 reps on your right side to complete 1 set.

Minna Says
You are not your circumstances but your possibilities. And your possibilities are endless.

FOCUS ON FORM

✤ Contract your abdominals to keep your back from sagging.
✤ Keep your shoulders down and away from your ears.
✤ As you walk your feet, avoid twisting or turning your body.

AT HOME/AT THE GYM

AT HOME: Instead of walking your feet, "jump" your feet apart. Then "jump" your feet back together. While you jump, make sure you maintain the contraction in your abs to protect your back.
AT THE GYM: Place your forearms on a Bosu ball, then perform the basic move as described.

BEGINNER

If this move proves too challenging, simply hold the Modified Plank position with your feet together for 10 to 30 seconds for each set.

INTERMEDIATE

Try to increase the speed at which you "walk" without compromising proper form.

ADVANCED

Instead of starting in the Modified Plank position (with your forearms on the floor), begin in the Full Plank position (arms extended and hands on the floor, wrists directly beneath your shoulders). Walk outward with your left foot and left hand at the same time. Repeat with your right foot and right hand. Return your left foot and hand to the starting position; repeat with your right foot and hand. Perform 5 to 10 repetitions leading with your left, then 5 to 10 leading with your right.

ORIGINAL MOVE

ADVANCED MOVE

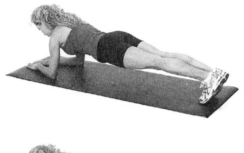

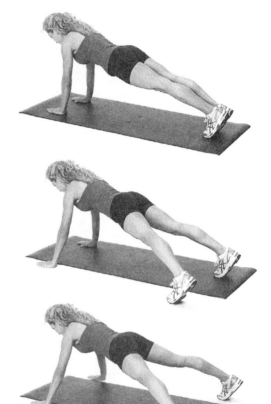

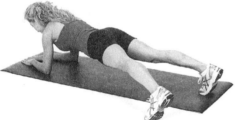

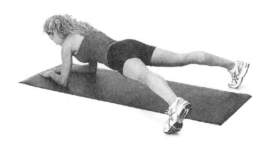

USE YOUR HEAD

The key to this move is to keep your body stable and to form one long line from your head to your heels. Whether you are holding the plank or moving your legs, picture your body as a long steel rod.

BREATHWORK

Breathe deeply and steadily through your nose throughout the move. Shallow breathing will make you fatigue more quickly.

SUGGESTED STRETCH

Static:
Cobra Pose
(page 32)
Moving Flexibility:
Child's Pose with Reach Across
(page 42)

✤ DIPPING TOES IN WATER

This small move will have a big impact on your abs. It strengthens the abdominal and core muscles.

SETS AND REPS

BEGINNER: 1 to 2 sets, 8 to 12 repetitions
INTERMEDIATE: 2 to 3 sets,
8 to 12 repetitions
ADVANCED: 3 sets, 8 to 12 repetitions

STARTING POSITION

Lie on your back with your arms at your sides and your palms flat on the floor. Lift your feet off the floor and bend your knees to 90 degrees so that they are over your hips. Contract your abdominals and draw your navel toward your spine.

THE MOVE

Keeping your knees bent and your abdominals tightly contracted, lower your toes toward the floor. Using your abdominal muscles, return your legs to the starting position to complete 1 repetition. Repeat until you complete 1 set.

FOCUS ON FORM

✤ To protect your lower back, maintain a constant contraction in your abdominals and keep your navel drawn toward your spine.

✤ It's okay to have a little space between the floor and the small of your back, but avoid excessively arching your back.

✤ Use your abdominal muscles to lower and lift your legs. Avoid pressing into the floor with your palms.

AT HOME/AT THE GYM

AT HOME: Perform the move as described above. If you own a stability ball, try the move below.

AT THE GYM: Hold a stability ball between your legs when you perform the move.

BEGINNER

Instead of lowering both legs at the same time, lower your right leg while keeping your left knee over your left hip. Return your right leg to the starting position and then lower your left leg, keeping your right knee over your right hip. Continue to alternate legs with each repetition until you complete 1 set.

INTERMEDIATE

Perform the move with your hands behind your head and your fingers touching but not interlaced. Also, lift your head and shoulders off the floor as you keep your abdominals tight.

ADVANCED

Perform the Intermediate move, but extend your arms and place them above your head, alongside your ears.

ORIGINAL MOVE

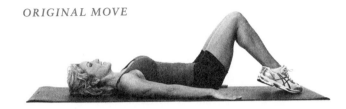

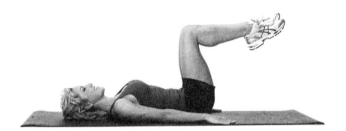

Minna Says
How and when you start aren't important, as long as you finish what you start.

ADVANCED MOVE

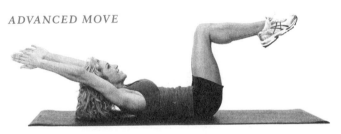

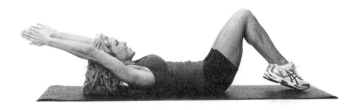

USE YOUR HEAD
As the move's name suggests, visualize yourself *slowly* dipping your toes into water, then *slowly* pulling them out.

BREATHWORK
Exhale as you lower your toes toward the floor. Inhale as you return to the starting position.

SUGGESTED STRETCH
Static:
Cobra Pose (page 32)
Moving Flexibility:
Kneeling Lunge (page 35)

✿ SUPERMAN

This move is a must for maintaining a strong core and healthy back. It not only strengthens the abdominal and lower back muscles, it also helps to improve posture.

SETS AND REPS

BEGINNER: 1 to 2 sets, 16 to 24 alternating repetitions with optional leg lifts (see opposite page)
INTERMEDIATE: 2 to 3 sets, 16 to 24 alternating repetitions
ADVANCED: 3 sets, 8 to 12 repetitions per side (see opposite page)

STARTING POSITION

You'll want to use a small folded towel or mat for this move. Lie on your belly with your arms stretched above your head alongside your ears (like Superman flies) and your palms flat on the floor. Spread your legs hip-width apart, with the soles of your feet pointed toward the ceiling. Place your forehead on the floor, using the towel or mat for comfort.

THE MOVE

Raise your right arm and left leg off the floor without twisting your body or shrugging your shoulders. Return to the starting position and repeat with your left arm and right leg. Continue to alternate sides until you complete 1 set.

Minna Says
We are all given possibilities. What we do with them determines who we are and who we will become.

FOCUS ON FORM

✿ Keep your shoulders down and away from your ears.
✿ Lift your arm and leg as high as you can without sacrificing comfort or form.
✿ Keep the arm and leg you are lifting straight. If your elbow or knee bends, you are lifting too high.

AT HOME/AT THE GYM

AT HOME: Lift and rotate your torso. From the starting position, place your arms along your sides with your palms flat on the floor. Space your legs hip-width apart. Keeping your head and spine aligned, lift your torso off the floor and reach back with your right hand, using an upward and turning motion as if you are reaching for something behind you. Return to the starting position.

AT THE GYM: Try a variation of this move on a stability ball. Lie belly-down on the ball with your feet on the floor and your toes turned inward. Place your hands behind your head with your fingertips touching, or allow your arms to hang off the sides of the ball. Lift your torso as high as you can while maintaining balance and proper form, then return to the starting position. Exhale as you lift, inhale as you lower.

BEGINNER

To reduce the intensity of the move, lift your leg, but keep both arms on the floor above your head. Alternate legs with each repetition until you complete 1 set.

INTERMEDIATE

Perform a "Swimming Superman": From the starting position, lift your right arm and left leg. As you lower them, immediately lift your left arm and right leg, as if you are swimming. Continue to alternate your arms and legs without pausing until you complete 1 set. Try to keep your arm and leg off the floor between repetitions, balancing only on your torso.

ADVANCED

Get on all fours and elongate your spine from your head to your tailbone. Extend your right arm and left leg, touching your fingertips and toes to the floor. From this position, lift and lower your right arm and left leg. Repeat, switching sides halfway through each set.

ORIGINAL MOVE

ADVANCED MOVE

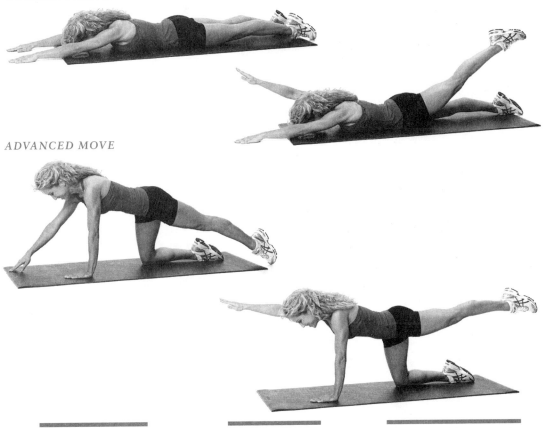

USE YOUR HEAD

Look! Up in the sky! There's no better visual for this move than Superman flying.

BREATHWORK

Exhale as you lift your arm and leg. Inhale as you lower them.

SUGGESTED STRETCH

Static:
Child's Pose with Reach Across
(page 30)

ROLL-UP

This mat move is such a challenge, you only need to do a few! It flattens and strengthens the abdominals, especially the rectus abdominis and transversus abdominis, and increases flexibility in the hamstrings and back.

SETS AND REPS

BEGINNER: 1 to 2 sets, 3 to 6 repetitions
INTERMEDIATE: 2 to 3 sets,
3 to 6 repetitions
ADVANCED: 2 to 3 sets, 3 to 6 repetitions

STARTING POSITION

On a mat, lie on your back with your legs straight and your arms extended above your head alongside your ears. Draw your navel toward your spine.

THE MOVE

Keeping your arms straight, raise them into the air over your head and then reach for your toes, tucking your chin into your chest and slowly curling your upper body toward your feet. Keep a deep curve in your abdominals and round your back all the way to the top of the move. Exhale and slowly return to the starting position, one vertebra at a time, until your body is flat on the floor.

FOCUS ON FORM

* Keep your chin tucked in, your abdominals in a deep curve, and your back rounded.
* As you roll up, squeeze your thighs together to help keep your feet and legs on the floor.
* Tuck your tailbone under and slowly return to the starting position, maintaining the curve in your upper body.

AT HOME/AT THE GYM

AT HOME: Try the roll-over. Assume the starting position, but place your arms by your sides, with your palms flat on the floor. Raise your legs straight up, point your toes toward the ceiling, then turn your feet outward. Use your abdominals to pull your thighs over your rib cage. (If you can, roll over onto the top of your shoulders and touch your toes to the floor behind your head.) Then, open your legs to the width of your shoulders, flex your feet by bringing your toes back toward your shin, and roll back to the starting position, one vertebra at a time.

AT THE GYM: For a mega-challenge, try this move while holding a 3-pound medicine ball.

BEGINNER

Perform a half roll-back: Sit tall on your sit bones on the floor. Align your hips and shoulders and extend your arms in front of you, palms down. Either extend your legs (most challenging) or bend your knees and place your feet flat on the floor (least challenging). Draw your navel toward your spine, curve your abdominals into a C-curve, and lower your torso backward toward the floor. When you get halfway to the floor, inhale and roll back up to the starting position, keeping a deep curve in your abdominals and rounding your back.

INTERMEDIATE

Grasp the ends of a short towel—one short enough to keep your wrists in line with your shoulders. This makes it much harder to cheat.

ADVANCED

Perfect your form. Focus on maintaining that deep abdominal curve and performing the move with fluidity and grace.

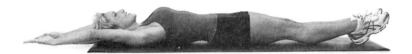

ORIGINAL MOVE

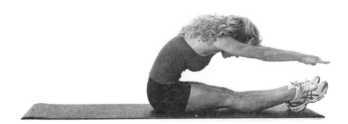

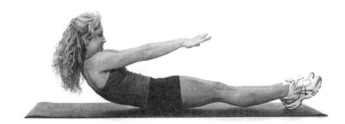

USE YOUR HEAD

Think of your body as a flat bumper sticker at the start of the move. As you roll up, slowly "peel off" the floor into a curve.

SUGGESTED STRETCH

Static:
Cobra Pose (page 32)
Moving Flexibility:
Kneeling Lunge (page 35)

Minna Says
Challenges are like dumbbells: They may be uncomfortable at first, but ultimately they make you stronger.

ROLL BACK AND REACH

This Pilates-based move helps build a sleek, sexy bikini tummy.
It tones and flattens the abdominals and strengthens the core.

SETS AND REPS

BEGINNER: 1 to 2 sets,
16 to 24 alternating repetitions
INTERMEDIATE: 2 to 3 sets,
16 to 24 alternating repetitions
ADVANCED: 3 sets,
16 to 24 alternating repetitions

STARTING POSITION

Sit tall on your sit bones on the floor, knees bent and feet flat on the floor about 2 feet beyond your bottom. Align your shoulders and hips. Extend your arms over your knees at shoulder height with your palms facing the floor. Contract your abdominals and pull your navel toward your spine.

THE MOVE

Shift your pelvis forward underneath you and round your abdominals so that your body is in a C-curve from the top of your head to the base of your spine. Leaning back, lower your torso halfway to the floor. As you hold the C-curve, rotate your trunk and sweep your left arm to the side, as if you are reaching for something behind you. Leave your right arm poised over your right knee. Keeping your abs tight and still holding the C-curve, sweep your left arm back to its starting position at shoulder height. Raise your torso to the starting position and realign your shoulders and hips. Repeat, alternating arms with every repetition until you complete 1 set.

FOCUS ON FORM

❖ Hold the C-curve position throughout the move.
❖ Keep your shoulders down and away from your ears.
❖ Rotate your trunk as far as you can while still contracting your abdominal muscles.

AT HOME/AT THE GYM

AT HOME: Perform the "At the Gym" move described below while holding a thick book, such as a dictionary, rather than a medicine ball.

AT THE GYM: Hold a medicine ball with both hands in front of you and assume the starting position. Lower your torso into a C-curve. Rotate to the left, moving the ball to or past your left hip. Return to the center and rotate to the right, moving the ball to or past your right hip, in one fluid motion. Continue to rotate from left to right until you complete 1 set. After the last repetition, still holding the ball in front of you and maintaining the C-curve, raise your torso to the starting position and realign your shoulders and hips.

BEGINNER

To lessen the intensity of the move, lightly hold the backs of your thighs rather than extending your arms. As you lower your torso, remove your left hand, sweep your arm backward and rotate your trunk, then return your hand to the back of your left thigh. Return to the starting position and repeat on the right side.

INTERMEDIATE

Try to sweep your arm further back and rotate your trunk in a greater arc while still maintaining correct form.

ADVANCED

Add a leg extension to the move: As you sweep your left arm backward and rotate your trunk, straighten and lift your left leg toward the ceiling, keeping your knees close together. Lower your leg as you rotate your trunk back to center and raise your torso into the starting position.

Minna Says
Don't put off a workout until tomorrow when you can do it today. Procrastination is the enemy of opportunity.

ORIGINAL MOVE

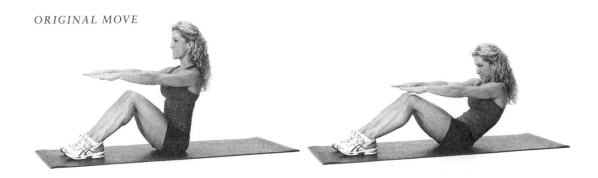

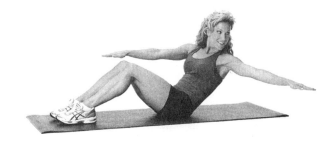

USE YOUR HEAD

This move is about maintaining that C-curve. Throughout the move, visualize the letter C and try to replicate its curve with your body.

BREATHWORK

Inhale at the top of the move. Exhale as you lower your torso and reach behind you. Inhale again as you realign your shoulders and hips.

SUGGESTED STRETCH

Moving Flexibility:
Lunge with One-Arm Reach
(page 43)

♣ BALLERINA TWIST

This fun move is a fusion of Pilates and ballet. It strengthens the rectus abdominis, transversus abdominis, and obliques; flattens the abdominals; and improves balance.

SETS AND REPS

BEGINNER: 1 to 2 sets, 12 to 20 alternating repetitions
INTERMEDIATE: 2 to 3 sets, 12 to 20 alternating repetitions
ADVANCED: 3 sets, 12 to 20 alternating repetitions

STARTING POSITION

Lie on your back on the floor with your body extended in one long, straight line. Turn your toes outward and squeeze your thighs together. Raise your arms into the air over your head and curve them slightly, like a ballerina's, with your fingertips pointing toward each other.

THE MOVE

Keeping your left arm in its curved position over your head, use your abdominals to lift and twist your torso to the right. As you lift and twist, lower your right forearm, still extended above your head, to the floor to slightly assist you. Return to the starting position and raise your right arm over your head. Now, lift and twist your torso to the left. As you lift and twist, keep your right arm raised over your head and lower your left forearm to the floor to slightly assist you. Alternate sides with each repetition until you complete 1 set.

Minna Says
Don't be afraid to be yourself. In fact, dare to be yourself.

FOCUS ON FORM

❖ Before you begin the move, draw your navel in toward your spine.
❖ Note that your abdominal muscles initiate the move. Rather than propping yourself up with your forearm, lift your torso with your abs.
❖ Keep your spine long. Reach with the fingertips of the arm over your head as you contract the abdominals on the opposite side to twist your body.
❖ Keep your shoulders down and away from your ears.
❖ Squeeze your inner thighs together throughout the move.

AT HOME/AT THE GYM

AT HOME: Perform a classical ballet move—*changement de pieds* (change of feet)—as you work your abdominals. From the starting position, raise your legs into the air so that they are perpendicular to the floor, over your hips. Contract your abdominals and lift your head, neck, and shoulders off the floor. Point and turn your toes outward, then place the outside edge of your right foot on the arch of your left foot. Then switch, placing the edge of your left foot on the arch of your right foot. As you switch feet, keep your legs together and contract your inner thighs. Perform 16 to 24 alternating reps.

AT THE GYM: Try this move on the stability ball. Place your neck, shoulders, and upper back on the ball, with your hips hanging off of it. Bend your knees and place your feet flat on the floor. Perform the move.

BEGINNER

Modify the starting position: Lie propped up on your forearms, with your palms flat on the floor and your fingertips facing forward. Leaving your right forearm on the floor, raise your left arm up and over as you twist to the right. Return to the starting position on both fore-arms and repeat, raising your right arm and twisting to the left.

INTERMEDIATE

Add a single-leg raise to the unmodified move. As you lift and twist to the right, with your left arm still raised over your head, lift your right leg off the floor to 45 degrees. Lower your leg and repeat, alternating sides, until you complete 1 set.

ADVANCED

Hold a 45-degree double-leg raise. From the starting position, lift both legs (in the toes-turned-out position) to a 45-degree angle. Just holding this position is a challenge. Remember to keep your abdominals tight as you twist your upper body. Return to the starting position, then twist to alternating sides until you complete 1 set.

ORIGINAL MOVE

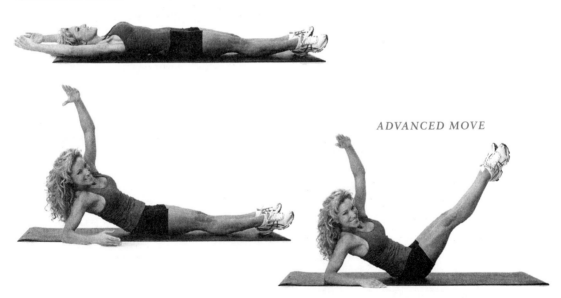

ADVANCED MOVE

USE YOUR HEAD
Picture yourself as a ballerina lying in bed in the starting position. Then, with one arm, reach over and up to turn off your bedside lamp before drifting off to sleep.

BREATHWORK
Exhale as you lift and twist your torso. Inhale as you return to the starting position.

SUGGESTED STRETCH
Moving Flexibility:
Child's Pose to Upward-Facing Dog
(page 44)

BICYCLE

Get those legs pumping! A scientific study rated this move number 1 in a list of the 13 most effective abdominal exercises. It strengthens the rectus abdominis and oblique muscles.

SETS AND REPS

BEGINNER: 1 to 2 sets,
16 to 24 alternating repetitions
INTERMEDIATE: 2 to 3 sets,
16 to 24 alternating repetitions
ADVANCED: 3 sets,
16 to 24 alternating repetitions

STARTING POSITION

Lie on your back with your knees bent and your feet flat on the floor. Place your hands behind your head with your fingers touching but not interlaced. Use your abdominals to lift your head, neck, and shoulders off the floor. Lift your legs and bend your knees to about a 90-degree angle, so that your knees are over your hips and your lower legs are parallel with floor.

THE MOVE

Slowly move your legs in a circle as though you are pedaling a bicycle, bending one leg as you extend the opposite leg. Twist and lift your torso, bringing your left shoulder up toward your right knee, then lifting your right shoulder toward your left knee. Extend each leg fully during every repetition. Continue, alternating sides on every repetition, until you complete 1 set.

> **Minna Says**
> To follow your dream, take one step at a time and, despite the challenges, never look back.

FOCUS ON FORM

* Perform the move slowly and with control.
* Contract your abdominal muscles as hard as you can and twist your torso as far as you can while still maintaining proper form.
* Avoid arching your back as you extend your legs to "pedal."
* Keep the movement fluid—no stopping as you alternate sides.

AT HOME/AT THE GYM

AT HOME: Perform a Modified Plank hold with a knee pull. Start in the Modified Plank hold position (see page 76). Pull your right knee toward your left hip bone, then straighten and extend your right leg behind you. Repeat with the left leg, pulling your left knee toward your right hip bone, then straightening and extending your left leg. Continue, alternating sides with each repetition, until you complete 1 set.

AT THE GYM: Hold a medicine ball as you lie with your back and shoulders on a stability ball, your feet flat on the floor and your knees bent. With both hands, lift the medicine ball over your head and look at it. Contract your abdominal muscles. Then, twist your torso to the right and lower the medicine ball as far to the right as you can without losing your balance. Then, lift the ball overhead again and twist to the left, lowering the medicine ball to the left. Continue to alternate twists until you complete 1 set. Beginners, perform this move without the medicine ball. When lifting your arms, press your palms together.

BEGINNER
Practice each part of the move separately. First, practice just the twisting motion without pedaling your legs. Then, practice pedaling, but don't twist. Tightly contract your abdominals throughout the move.

INTERMEDIATE
Work toward lowering your legs closer to the floor, contracting your abdominals tightly. The more you lower your legs, the more challenging the move becomes.

ADVANCED
To challenge your abs even more, perform the move with both legs extended straight out, and stretching them back over your head, alternating them one at a time.

ORIGINAL MOVE

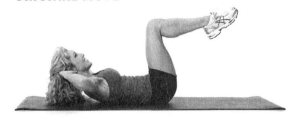

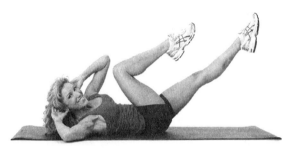

ADVANCED MOVE

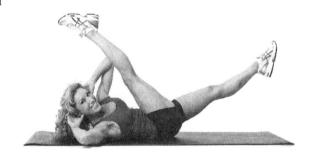

USE YOUR HEAD
Picture yourself on a bicycle. To keep your balance, you must keep your abs contracted. If you relax them, you'll lose your balance. *Remember:* Your abs power the move. Your legs just go along for the ride.

BREATHWORK
Inhale and exhale through your nose throughout the move. Avoid holding your breath.

SUGGESTED STRETCH
Moving Flexibility:
Child's Pose to Upward-Facing Dog
(page 44)

6

BIKINI BELLY
MASTER

If you've mastered the Skilled Bikini Belly moves, these push-you-to-the-limit abdominal and core exercises will further define your midsection, increase your core strength, and challenge your balance and coordination.

These fun, funky moves aren't the same old, same old. Because they target your core from every angle, they will improve your performance in other types of physical activity, such as skiing or biking, and allow you to wear any body-hugging fashion with confidence. You'll need a towel or mat, plus a Bosu and/or a stability ball if you want to perform the variations in the "At the Gym" sections.

FEATURED EXERCISES:

♣SCISSORS

♣ORIGAMI CRUNCH

♣SIDE PLANK

♣GYMNAST ABS

♣ARM AND LEG EXTENSION

♣REVERSE PLANK

♣KNEE DROP

♣TWIST AND DROP

✤

SCISSORS

This Pilates-based move will firm and flatten your entire midsection. It strengthens the rectus abdominis, obliques, and transversus abdominis (the muscle that holds in your stomach).

SETS AND REPS

BEGINNER: 1 to 2 sets,
16 to 24 alternating repetitions
INTERMEDIATE: 2 to 3 sets,
16 to 24 alternating repetitions
ADVANCED: 3 sets,
16 to 24 alternating repetitions

STARTING POSITION

Lie on your back on the floor, arms at your sides with your palms down. Bring your knees toward your chest and draw your navel toward your spine. Press your legs and feet together and extend them, toes pointed, toward the ceiling. Inhale deeply, then exhale and lift your torso until your shoulder blades leave the floor. As you do this, reach with outstretched arms for your calves and draw your shoulders down and back.

THE MOVE

Keeping your legs and back elongated, inhale. Then exhale as you raise your still-straightened right leg over your chest and reach with both hands for your right calf. At the same time, lower your left leg as far as you can without losing form or touching the ground. Keeping your chest lifted, inhale. Exhale as you lower your right leg toward the floor. At the same time, lift your left leg toward your chest, reaching with both hands for your left calf. Continue to alternate legs until you complete 1 set.

Minna Says
You can't sail new seas if you fear losing sight of the shore.

FOCUS ON FORM

✤ Bring your leg toward your chest as far as you comfortably can with good form.

✤ Lower your leg toward the floor as far as you comfortably can without losing the contraction in your abdominals. If you cannot hold the contraction, you may strain your lower back.

✤ Stabilize your pelvis by drawing in your abdominals throughout the move.

AT HOME/AT THE GYM

AT HOME: Perform the move as described above. If you own a Bosu ball, try the variation below.

AT THE GYM: Beginners, you can try the Intermediate/Advanced move, opposite, but do it on the floor. Intermediate and advanced readers, try a bicycle version of this move on a Bosu ball. Lie faceup on the ball so that the small of your back is on the ball and your legs are extended in front of you. Contract your abdominals and lift your shoulders off the ball. Bend your right knee and bring it toward your chest, grasping it lightly with both hands. Switch legs; repeat until you complete 1 set. Work toward keeping your straight leg off the floor so that your entire body is balanced on the ball.

BEGINNER

Perform the bicycle move described in "At the Gym" on the floor. Try to keep your straight leg off the floor.

INTERMEDIATE

For an increased challenge, try spreading your arms out perpendicularly to your body.

ADVANCED

Move your arms with your legs: As you bring your right leg toward your chest, straighten your right arm and bring it along with your leg. Repeat with your left arm and left leg.

ORIGINAL MOVE

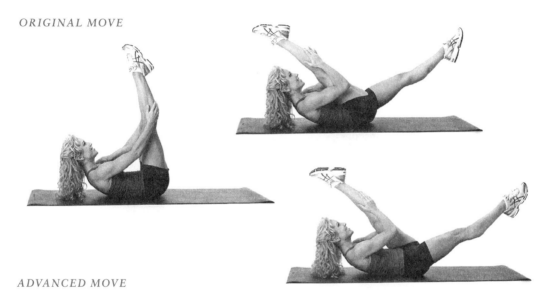

ADVANCED MOVE

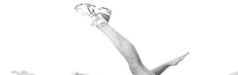

USE YOUR HEAD

Picture your legs as a pair of scissors opening and closing. Your core, like the hand holding the scissors, stays immobile.

BREATHWORK

Exhale as you raise your leg over your chest. Inhale as you switch legs.

SUGGESTED STRETCH

Static:
Cobra Pose (page 32)
Moving Flexibility:
Kneeling Lunge (page 35)

✤ ORIGAMI CRUNCH

*This move improves core strength and endurance
and flattens, tones, and defines the abdominal muscles.*

SETS AND REPS

BEGINNER: 1 to 2 sets, 8 to 12 repetitions
INTERMEDIATE: 2 to 3 sets,
8 to 12 repetitions
ADVANCED: 3 sets, 8 to 12 repetitions

STARTING POSITION

Lie on your back with your arms at your
sides, your knees bent, and your feet flat
on the floor. Contract your abdominals to
draw your navel toward your spine. Lifting your feet, bend your knees to 90
degrees and raise them over your hips so
your lower legs are parallel with the floor
and your toes are pointed. Rest your
palms lightly on your knees. Use your
abdominal muscles to lift your head, neck,
and shoulders off the floor.

THE MOVE

While contracting your abdominals,
"unfold" yourself by straightening and
extending your legs and arms. Hold your
legs at a 45-degree angle and straighten
your arms alongside your ears, but keep
your head and shoulders off the floor.
"Fold up" by returning to the starting
position. Repeat until you complete 1 set.

FOCUS ON FORM

✤ To maintain your balance, contract
your abdominals tightly and keep your
navel drawn toward your spine.

AT HOME/AT THE GYM

AT HOME: Sit at the edge of a sturdy
bench or chair. Hold the edge of the seat
and tuck your knees in toward your chest.
Find your balance, then extend and lower
your legs without allowing your toes to
touch the floor. Use your abdominals to
tuck your bent knees toward your chest.
Repeat until you complete 1 set.
AT THE GYM: Test your core strength and
balance by simply holding the starting
position on the round side of a Bosu ball.
Hold for 10 to 30 seconds, breathing
deeply.

BEGINNER

If extending both your arms and your legs
proves too challenging, extend only your
legs. Wrap your arms around your thighs
so that your palms are on the backs of
your thighs, then straighten your legs to a
45-degree angle.

INTERMEDIATE

After you unfold your arms and legs, hold
for a count of three. Then return to the
starting position.

ADVANCED

Perform the Intermediate move as described above and add a reverse crunch.
Perform the move. As you return to the
starting position, use your abdominals to
lift your pelvis off the floor, then lower it
into the starting position.

ORIGINAL MOVE

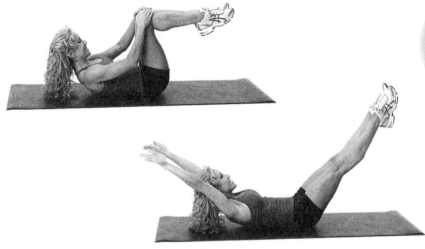

Minna Says
When you have faith, you can see the invisible and achieve the impossible.

ADVANCED MOVE

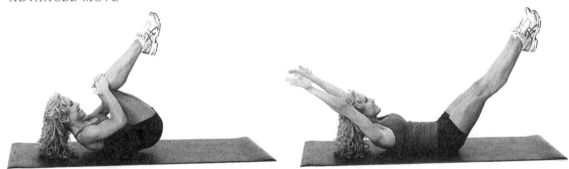

USE YOUR HEAD

Origami is the Japanese art of folding paper into decorative shapes. Picture yourself as a beautiful work of origami as you fold and unfold from your core.

BREATHWORK

Exhale as you extend your arms and legs. Inhale as you return to the starting position.

SUGGESTED STRETCH

Moving Flexibility:
Lunge with
One-Arm Reach
(page 43)

SIDE PLANK

This move will allow you to slip into that body-hugging cocktail dress. It strengthens the rectus abdominis, transversus abdominis, and obliques. It also tones the arms, shoulders, and legs and improves balance.

SETS AND REPS

BEGINNER: 1 to 2 sets, holding the modified position for 10 to 30 seconds per side (see below)

INTERMEDIATE: 2 to 3 sets, holding the full position for 15 to 30 seconds per side

ADVANCED: 2 to 3 sets, holding the full position for 15 to 30 seconds per side and adding a leg raise (see opposite page)

STARTING POSITION

Start in the Front Plank position (see page 90). Essentially, the Front Plank is the top of a pushup—arms straight, wrists beneath the shoulders, legs extended, and toes on the floor. Your body should form one long, straight line from your head to your heels. Contract your abdominal muscles.

THE MOVE

Now, move into the Side Plank. Bring your right hand to the center, halfway between its starting position and your left hand. Start to turn your body to the left, shifting your weight from your toes to the outer side of your right foot and stacking your left foot on top of your right. Lift your left arm off the floor. Finally, extend your left arm toward the ceiling, in line with your shoulders. Your body should form one long, straight line from your head to your feet, sideways. Look straight ahead and hold this position for the length of time recommended for your experience level, then switch sides and repeat to complete the set.

FOCUS ON FORM

❖ Contract your abdominal muscles tightly throughout the move, keeping your navel drawn toward your spine.

❖ Squeeze your shoulder blades together to pull your shoulders back and down.

❖ Contract the triceps of the supporting arm throughout the move.

AT HOME/AT THE GYM

AT HOME: Try a Side Plank twist. Perform the Intermediate move as described. Instead of holding the position, however, lower your left arm, twist your torso, and reach for your right hip. Try to stretch your left hand past your right hip. Then, untwist your torso and return to the starting position. Repeat until you complete 5 to 10 repetitions, then switch sides.

AT THE GYM: Perform the move with your supporting hand on a Bosu ball.

BEGINNER

To perform a modified version of this move until you gain strength and balance, assume the starting position, but bend your right knee and place it on the floor beneath your right hip. Or, perform the move while pressing the soles of your feet against a wall for balance.

INTERMEDIATE

To challenge your stability even more, turn your head and look at your left hand as your left arm is raised above your head.

ADVANCED

Perform the move and raise your top (left) leg as high as you can. Keep your toes pointed forward and your hips and shoulders squared. Or, perform 6 to 12 leg lifts as you hold the move, then switch sides.

ORIGINAL MOVE

ADVANCED MOVE

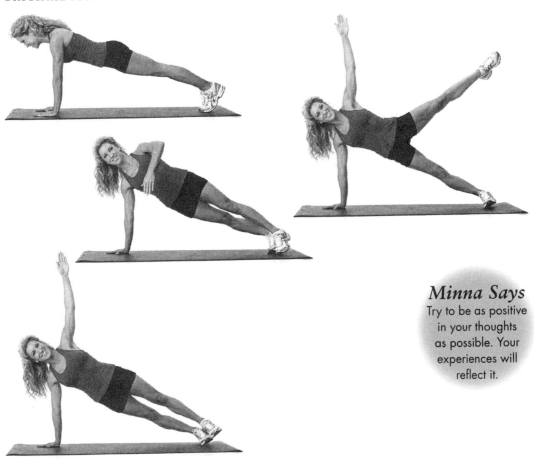

Minna Says
Try to be as positive in your thoughts as possible. Your experiences will reflect it.

USE YOUR HEAD
If you have ever seen the circus troupe Cirque du Soleil, you know that the body truly is an amazing machine. Perform this move slowly and carefully, drawing inspiration from the strength, power, and beauty of the performers' acrobatic feats.

BREATHWORK
Inhale and exhale deeply and steadily through your nose, letting the air hit the back of your throat.

SUGGESTED STRETCH
Static:
Child's Pose with Reach Across
(page 30)

GYMNAST ABS

This move—a conditioning drill often used by gymnasts, who have cores of steel—will tighten your abs, too. It also works your chest, shoulder, and triceps muscles.

SETS AND REPS

BEGINNER: 1 to 2 sets, 8 to 12 repetitions
INTERMEDIATE: 2 to 3 sets,
8 to 12 repetitions
ADVANCED: 3 sets, 8 to 12 repetitions,
or 15 to 30 seconds (see opposite page)

STARTING POSITION

Roll up a towel or mat. Sit on it and grasp it with your palms down and fingers pointing forward. Extend your legs straight out in front of you with your feet together, knees straight, and heels only on the floor. Contract your abdominal muscles and draw your navel toward your spine.

THE MOVE

Straighten your arms and lift your backside off the floor, supporting yourself with only your heels and hands. Lower your chin slightly as you try to push your hips and bottom behind your arms. Hold for a count of three (if you can!) and return to the starting position. Repeat until you complete 1 set.

> *Minna Says*
> Your options are limited only by your fears.

FOCUS ON FORM

♣ Concentrate on pulling in your navel and strongly contracting your abs.
♣ Keep your shoulders down and away from your ears.

AT HOME/AT THE GYM

AT HOME: Beginners, assume the starting position, but spread your legs so that your feet are 2 to 3 feet apart. Intermediate and advanced readers, place your hands between your legs with your palms down and your index fingers and thumbs touching and try to lift your backside off the floor.

AT THE GYM: Beginners, perform tucks while sitting on the floor. Sit tall on your sit bones with your palms flat on the floor at your sides and your legs extended in front of you with your heels on the floor. Bend your knees and tuck them toward your chest, lifting your heels off the floor. Return to the starting position. Intermediate and advanced readers, perform leg raises as you hang on a bar. Ask a trainer to help you get onto the bar and keep your body still for each repetition. As you hang from your hands on the bar, lift your legs as high as you can—either with your knees bent (easiest) or straight (most challenging)—without using momentum or swinging your legs. Slowly return to the starting position.

BEGINNER

To make the move less challenging, sit on the bottom step of a staircase with your palms flat on the step, so that your legs are lower than your torso. It's easier to lift your bottom when your legs are lower than your hips.

INTERMEDIATE

As you perform the move, try to lift one leg off the floor. Alternate legs with each repetition.

ORIGINAL MOVE

ADVANCED

Try to hold the position for longer and longer periods, up to 30 seconds. For the ultimate challenge, try to lift your legs straight off the floor and balance your body on your hands. If you can do it, congratulations! You've just performed the pike position press, a classic gymnast's move.

ADVANCED MOVE

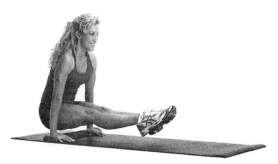

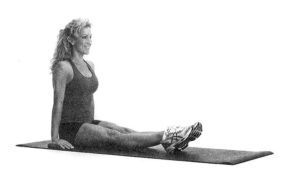

USE YOUR HEAD

The abdominals power this move. As you contract your abs to lift your bottom off the floor, picture your rib cage meeting your hip bones.

BREATHWORK

Exhale as you lift your backside off the floor and push your hips and bottom backward. Inhale as you return to the starting position.

SUGGESTED STRETCH

Kneeling Lunge
(page 25)

ARM AND LEG EXTENSION

This move helps elongate your muscles so that you'll stand tall and pretty instead of slouching in that hot new outfit. It strengthens the core muscles and improves balance, coordination, and posture.

SETS AND REPS

BEGINNER: 1 to 2 sets, 8 to 12 repetitions
INTERMEDIATE: 2 to 3 sets,
8 to 12 repetitions
ADVANCED: 3 sets,
8 to 12 repetitions with arm and leg abduction (see below)

STARTING POSITION

Get down on all fours with your wrists beneath your shoulders and your knees beneath your hips. Contract your abdominal muscles and draw your navel toward your spine. Look at the floor. Your body should form one long, straight line from your head to your tailbone. Extend your right arm and left leg, letting your fingertips and toes touch the floor.

THE MOVE

Lift your right arm and left leg until they are parallel with the floor. Lower them to the starting position—keeping them straight!—until your fingertips and toes are just grazing the floor. Switch sides for your second set. If you're performing an odd number of sets, switch sides halfway through each set.

FOCUS ON FORM

✤ Keep the arm and leg you're lifting straight throughout the move. Bending your leg as you lower it allows your core muscles to rest.
✤ Distribute your weight evenly between the hand and knee on the floor.
✤ Maintain the contraction in your abdominals throughout the move.

AT HOME/AT THE GYM

AT HOME: Try the Swimming Superman move (see page 135).
AT THE GYM: Perform hyperextensions on a stability ball. Lie on the ball belly-down, so that your chest, abdomen, and hips are on the ball and your arms hang down on both sides. Hang your legs off the ball so that your toes touch the floor. Turn your toes inward to force your back, rather than your glutes, to do most of the work. Using your back muscles, lift your torso as high as you can while maintaining your balance. Return to the starting position. Repeat until you complete 1 set.

BEGINNER

If the move proves too challenging, lie on your stomach instead of balancing on one hand and one knee.

INTERMEDIATE

At the top of the move, when your arm and leg are parallel with the floor, hold for a count of three.

ADVANCED

Add arm and leg abduction: Perform the move as described. At the top of the move, rotate your arm and leg as far as possible out to the side, bring them back in, and return to the starting position. This variation is extremely challenging. Alternate sides with each repetition to make it less intense.

ORIGINAL MOVE

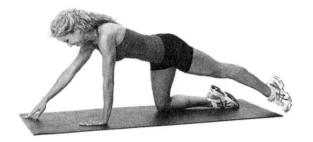

Minna Says
There is no elevator to success; you have to take the stairs. But you can certainly take them two at a time!

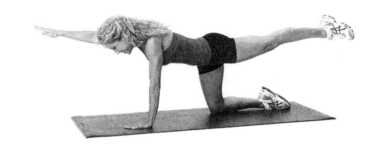

ADVANCED MOVE

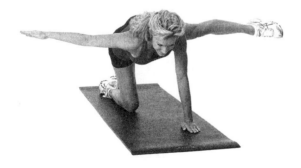

USE YOUR HEAD
Visualize yourself performing the move in a pool, working against the water's resistance.

BREATHWORK
Exhale as you lift your arm and leg. Inhale as you return to the starting position.

SUGGESTED STRETCH
Moving Flexibility:
Child's Pose with Reach Across (page 42)

REVERSE PLANK

This move is an extremely effective tummy-tightener. Besides strengthening the core muscles, it also tones the glutes and hamstrings and increases flexibility in the shoulders and biceps.

SETS AND REPS

BEGINNER: 1 to 2 sets, holding for 10 to 20 seconds
INTERMEDIATE: 2 to 3 sets, holding for 15 to 30 seconds
ADVANCED: 3 sets, 6 to 10 leg walks per side (see opposite page)

STARTING POSITION

Sit tall on your sit bones. Extend your legs in front of you. Rest your hands—palms down and fingers pointing forward—by the sides of your bottom. Tighten your abdominal muscles and pull your shoulders back and down. Pressing your hands and heels into the floor and leaning back, lift your pelvis off the floor until your body forms one long line from your head to your heels.

THE MOVE

Hold this position for the length of time recommended for your fitness level. Concentrate on maintaining one long line.

FOCUS ON FORM

✤ Contract your abdominals tightly to keep that nice long line. Avoid letting your pelvis drop.
✤ Look at the ceiling to keep your head in line with your body.
✤ Squeeze your shoulder blades together to keep your shoulders back and down.

AT HOME/AT THE GYM

AT HOME: Perform a one-legged Bridge (see page 172). Lie on your back with your knees bent and your feet flat on the floor. Place your arms by your sides. Using your abdominal muscles and glutes, lift your pelvis until your body forms one long line from your knees to your shoulders. Extend and straighten your right leg and hold for 10 to 30 seconds or perform leg lifts by lowering your right leg, keeping your knee straight, until it is just above the floor and then lifting it back in line with your body. Switch sides, lifting up your left leg. Continue alternating leg lifts for a total of 10 to 12 alternating repetitions per set.
AT THE GYM: Try a straight-leg Bridge on a stability ball. Lie on your back with your feet on a stability ball and your knees soft. Use your glutes to lift your pelvis off the floor, then lower it again, supporting yourself on your shoulders. Repeat until you complete 1 set.

BEGINNER

Place your hands on the bottom step of a staircase and your feet on the floor. The extra height makes the move a bit easier.

INTERMEDIATE

If you are able to hold the position for the time indicated, test your stability: Softly rock from side to side, shifting your weight slightly to the right (so that your right hand and right foot bear more of your weight), then to the left. Repeat, performing the rocking motion for a total of 10 to 20 repetitions to complete the set.

ADVANCED

From the Reverse Plank position, perform leg walks: Walk your right foot to the right and then your left foot to the left, so that your feet are 1 to 3 feet apart. Then walk your right foot back to the starting position, followed by your left foot, so that your feet are together again. Avoid dropping your pelvis; maintain that nice long line.

Minna Says
The smallest action means as much as the greatest intention.

ORIGINAL MOVE

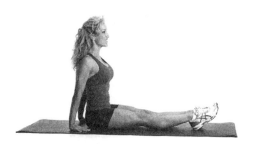

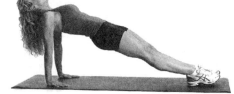

ADVANCED MOVE

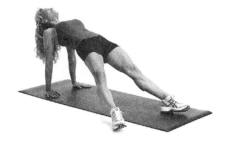

USE YOUR HEAD
Imagine that a rope tied around your pelvis is lifting it to keep your body in one unbroken line. Keep your abdominals and glutes tight—they act as the rope.

BREATHWORK
Breathe deeply and rhythmically through your nose.

SUGGESTED STRETCH
Static:
Seated Forward Bend
(page 23)
and Cobra Pose
(page 32)

✤ KNEE DROP

This move nips your waist and sculpts a taut, marvelous midriff. It tightens the rectus abdominis, strengthens the transversus abdominis, and tones the obliques.

SETS AND REPS

BEGINNER: 1 to 2 sets,
16 to 24 alternating repetitions
INTERMEDIATE: 2 to 3 sets,
16 to 24 alternating repetitions
with leg extension (see opposite page)
ADVANCED: 3 sets,
16 to 24 alternating repetitions with leg
extension and one-arm reach (see opposite
page)

STARTING POSITION

Lie on your back with your arms at your sides. Bend your knees and place your feet flat on the floor. Contract your abdominals and draw your navel toward your spine. Lift your legs off the floor and bend your knees to 90 degrees so that your knees are over your hips and your lower legs are parallel with the floor.

THE MOVE

Lower your knees as far to the right as you comfortably can with good form. Using your abdominal muscles, return to the starting position. Repeat, lowering your knees to the left. Continue, alternating sides with each repetition, until you complete 1 set.

FOCUS ON FORM

✤ To stabilize your body, contract your abdominals and draw your navel toward your spine.
✤ Avoid "cheating" by pressing your hands into the floor. Use your abs, rather than your triceps, to power the move.

✤ Keep your shoulders down and away from your ears.
✤ Keep your lower legs parallel to the floor and your knees over your hips.

AT HOME/AT THE GYM

AT HOME: Try the cancan extension (a Pilates move). Sit tall on the floor or on a mat with your arms extended behind you for support. Bend your knees, squeeze your thighs together, and bring your heels off the floor and close to your bottom, with your toes pointed and just grazing the floor. Lower your knees to the right, about halfway to the floor, so that your feet stay close to your bottom, then straighten your legs and lift them straight up. Return to the starting position. Switch sides, lowering your knees to the left.

AT THE GYM: Perform the move with the smallest stability ball positioned under your knees, resting against the back of your thighs.

BEGINNER

If you need help, enlist a wall. Assume the starting position, but place the soles of your feet on the wall so that your knees are bent at 90 degrees. To perform the move, walk your feet to the right. (Try to find a balance between using your abdominals and allowing your feet to assist.) Then walk them back to the starting position. Repeat, walking your feet to the left, then returning to the starting position. Continue, alternating sides with each repetition, until you complete 1 set.

INTERMEDIATE

Add a leg extension. Perform the move as described. After you lower your knees to the right, straighten your legs, bend your knees again, and return to the starting position. Repeat, lowering your knees to the left. Continue, alternating sides with each repetition, until you complete 1 set.

ADVANCED

Add a one-arm reach. Perform the Intermediate move as described. As you extend your legs to the right, crunch your abdominal muscles to lift your head, neck, and shoulders off the floor. Reach up and over with your left hand to try to touch your toes. Lower your head, neck, shoulders, and arm, bend your knees, and return to the starting position. Switch sides and alternate repetitions to complete 1 set.

ORIGINAL MOVE

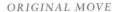

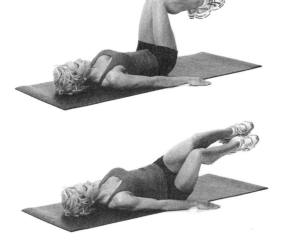

ADVANCED MOVE

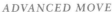

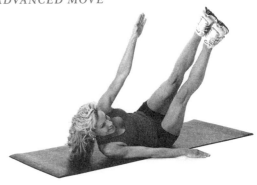

USE YOUR HEAD

Picture a child's punching bag, the kind that is filled with air and weighted at the bottom. When you punch it, the bag pops right back up again. Keep your core as stable as that bag, so that no matter how far your legs drop, you maintain your stability.

BREATHWORK

Exhale as you lower your knees to the side. Inhale as you return to the starting position.

SUGGESTED STRETCH

Static:
Spinal Twist
(page 31)

Minna Says
A bend in the road is not the end of the road unless you fail to make the turn.

TWIST AND DROP

A fusion of dance and gymnastics, this move is a unique way to develop abs of steel. It tones the rectus abdominis and obliques, strengthens the transversus abdominis, increases hamstring flexibility, and shapes the inner thighs.

SETS AND REPS

BEGINNER: 1 to 2 sets,
12 to 20 alternating repetitions
INTERMEDIATE: 2 to 3 sets,
12 to 20 alternating repetitions
ADVANCED: 3 sets,
12 to 20 alternating repetitions

STARTING POSITION

Stand with your feet slightly more than shoulder-width apart. Bend forward at the hips and place your hands flat on the floor, directly beneath your shoulders and at least 12 inches from your feet. (Since you're in a straddle position, your hands will not be in line with your feet.) Place your feet flat on the floor or raise your heels so that only your toes are touching the floor. Look at the floor. Draw your navel toward your spine.

THE MOVE

Using your abdominal muscles, lift your right foot off the floor. Keeping your right leg straight, sweep it across in front of your left foot. Twist your body and lower your hips toward the floor, so your left hip is facing the ceiling and your right hip is facing the floor. *Check your position:* Your left knee should be bent and you should be balancing on your hands, still in the starting position, and the toes of your left foot. Your right leg should

Minna Says
Never look back unless you're planning to go that way.

be straight, with your knee in front of your left foot. Look straight ahead. Using your abdominal muscles, untwist your body and return to the starting position. Switch sides, twisting and dropping to the right and sweeping with your left leg. Continue, alternating sides with each repetition, until you complete 1 set.

FOCUS ON FORM

✤ Use your abdominal muscles to initiate the movement.
✤ Contract your abdominals hard and draw your navel toward your spine.
✤ Keep your shoulders down and away from your ears.

AT HOME/AT THE GYM

AT HOME: Add an inner thigh lift at the bottom of the move (when your right leg is straight and in front of your left leg). As you hold this position, lift and lower your right leg to work your inner thigh and abs. Repeat to complete the set.

AT THE GYM: Place your hands on the flat side of a Bosu ball, then perform the move.

BEGINNER

Perform the move with your hands on the bottom step of a staircase.

INTERMEDIATE

At the bottom of the move, try to raise the knee of your front leg to meet the knee of your back leg.

ADVANCED

Add an arm raise. Perform the move as described. As you reach the bottom of the move (when your right leg is across your left), raise your left arm up until it points to the ceiling.

Then lower it as you untwist and return to the starting position. Switch sides, lifting your right arm as you cross your left leg in front of your right.

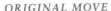

ORIGINAL MOVE

ADVANCED MOVE

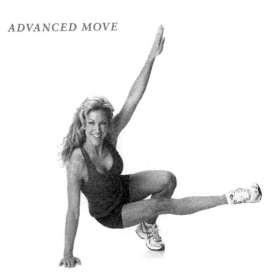

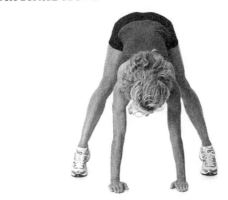

USE YOUR HEAD

If you're a little bawdy, you can picture this move as part of a striptease. In the starting position, your butt is in the air, and then you twist and drop to slide into a sexy floor pose.

BREATHWORK

Inhale before you perform the move. Exhale as you twist and drop. Inhale as you return to the starting position. Exhale as you switch sides.

SUGGESTED STRETCH
Static:
Kneeling Lunge
(page 25)
and Spinal Twist
(page 31)

PART 3

BOY SHORTS
Bottom

If you're less than happy with your butt, hips, or thighs, take heart: You can build a supple, jiggle-free lower body that is perfect for bikinis and boy shorts in as little as 4 weeks.

That's because the lower body's large muscles are quick to respond to TLC (tough love and cardio). The gluteal muscles, or glutes, include the gluteus maximus—the roundest part of the butt—and the lower buttocks. The thigh is composed of four major muscles. The quadriceps (quad) is located at the front of the thigh and the hamstring is in the back. The abductors are the muscles of the outer thigh, whereas the adductors are those of the inner thigh.

The moves in this section zero in on lower body trouble spots, helping to lift, shape, and sculpt. Along with regular cardio and a sensible, low-fat diet, performing these moves can make a significant difference in a surprisingly short time.

NOVICE

SQUAT

STEP-UP

HIP EXTENSION

BRIDGE

LEG LIFT

KNEE/HEEL TAP

LEG ABDUCTION

STATIONARY LUNGE

SKILLED

ALTERNATING
REVERSE LUNGE

CURTSY LUNGE

FROGGY
DOUBLE-LEG LIFT

SIDE LUNGE

PLIÉ SQUAT

STANDING
HIP EXTENSION

MASTER

DEAD LIFT

T POSE

SPLIT-LEG LUNGE

ONE-LEGGED SQUAT

REVERSE PLANK
WITH LEG LIFT

WALKING LUNGE

7

BOY SHORTS BOTTOM
NOVICE

If you're new to strength training, these basic but super-effective moves are the blocks you will use to build your lower body fitness program, and they will significantly trim and shape your hips, thighs, and butt in record time. To get the best results, combine these exercises with a healthy diet and at least 30 minutes of cardio on most or all days of the week. If you are working out at home, you will need a Bosu ball and/or a stability ball if you wish to try the variations in the "At the Gym" sections.

FEATURED EXERCISES:

♣SQUAT

♣STEP-UP

♣HIP EXTENSION

♣BRIDGE

♣LEG LIFT

♣KNEE/HEEL TAP

♣LEG ABDUCTION

♣STATIONARY LUNGE

♣ SQUAT

Boy shorts season comes and goes, but Squats keep your bottom tight and toned all year-round. This classic move builds and sculpts the glutes, tones the quadriceps, and improves balance.

SETS AND REPS

BEGINNER: 1 to 2 sets, 8 to 12 repetitions, no weight
INTERMEDIATE: 2 to 3 sets, 8 to 12 repetitions, 5- to 15-pound dumbbells
ADVANCED: 3 sets, 8 to 12 repetitions, 12- to 25-pound dumbbells

STARTING POSITION

Stand with your feet hip- or shoulder-width apart and your feet turned slightly outward. Hold the dumbbells at your sides with your palms facing inward. Contract your abdominal muscles, square your hips and shoulders, and draw your shoulders back and down.

THE MOVE

Push your hips backward as if you're going to sit in a chair, bend your knees, and lower into the Squat until your thighs are parallel with the floor. Slowly return to the starting position, using your glutes to lift your body, to complete 1 repetition.

FOCUS ON FORM ————

♣ Contract your abdominals throughout the move to support your lower back.
♣ To prevent knee injuries, keep your knees directly over your toes.
♣ Squat only until your thighs are parallel with the floor to protect your lower back.
♣ If your back rounds, arches, or feels strained or if your knees shake, you may be using too much weight.

AT HOME/AT THE GYM

AT HOME: Try a plyometric jump squat. Perform the first step of the move as directed. Then, instead of returning to the starting position, use your quadriceps and glutes to jump off the floor as high as you can. When you land, bend your knees and immediately lower into the Squat. Repeat until you complete 1 set.

AT THE GYM: If you are new to Squats, use a stability ball to perfect your form. Stand with your back to a wall with the ball between the wall and the small of your back. Then perform the move, rolling the ball along your spine toward your neck as you lower yourself.

BEGINNER

At first, place your hands on your hips as you perform this move. After you learn proper form, keep your arms at your sides, as if you were holding dumbbells. Remember to keep your shoulders back and down.

INTERMEDIATE

This variation, which is practice for a One-Legged Squat, targets the glutes even more. As you lower into the Squat, shift your weight onto one foot while keeping your hips and shoulders squared. Lower yourself until your thighs are parallel with the floor, then return to the starting position. On the next repetition, shift your weight to the other foot.

ADVANCED

Try the challenging One-Legged Squat (see page 204). Use no weights until you have mastered the form. Stand on one leg, lightly resting only the toes of your other foot on the floor. Lower yourself as far as you can while still maintaining your balance and correct form. Return to the starting position by pressing into your heel.

Minna Says
Be right here, right now. When you live in the moment, you can move mountains.

ORIGINAL MOVE

ADVANCED MOVE

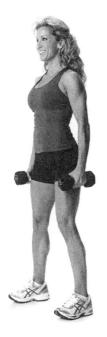 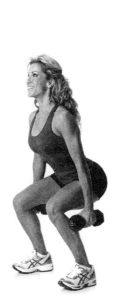 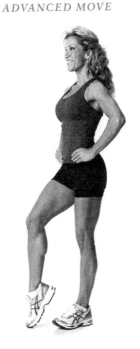 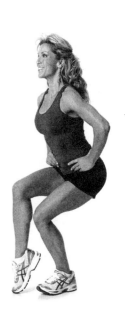

USE YOUR HEAD

Imagine an invisible string running through your body, the ends emerging from the top of your head and your tailbone. Pull up on the end coming from your head and down on the end coming from your tailbone.

BREATHWORK

Inhale as you lower yourself into the Squat. Exhale as you return to the starting position.

SUGGESTED STRETCH
Static:
Modified Hurdler
(page 27)
and/or Standing Quadriceps
(page 28)

STEP-UP

Step-ups target the "bottom line," shaping and lifting your backside. They shape and tone the glutes and provide some aerobic conditioning.

SETS AND REPS

BEGINNER: 1 to 2 sets,
8 to 12 repetitions per leg, no weight
INTERMEDIATE: 2 to 3 sets,
8 to 12 repetitions per leg,
5- to 12-pound dumbbells
ADVANCED: 3 sets,
8 to 12 repetitions per leg,
12- to 25-pound dumbbells

STARTING POSITION

Hold a dumbbell in each hand with your palms facing inward. Stand 1 to 2 feet in front of and facing a step bench, stair, or other sturdy platform with your feet hip-width apart. Contract your abdominal muscles and square your shoulders and hips.

THE MOVE

Step onto the bench with your right foot, transferring most of your weight to your heel. Bring your left foot onto the bench, too, to help you balance. Carefully step backward off the bench, starting with your left foot and following with your right. Repeat, always starting with your right foot, until you complete 8 to 12 reps, then switch sides so you are starting with your left foot.

FOCUS ON FORM

✤ Contract your abdominals throughout the move to protect your lower back.
✤ Keep your dumbbells at your sides. Swinging your arms will upset your balance.
✤ Keep the knee of the stepping leg directly over your foot.

AT HOME/AT THE GYM

AT HOME: Perform the move as described above. If you have a sturdy gym bench at home, try the move below.
AT THE GYM: Try the crisscross Step-up. While holding the dumbbells at your sides, stand beside a bench. First with your right foot and then with your left, step up onto the bench. Next, cross your left leg behind your right and lower your left foot to the floor. Keep your right foot on the bench. Use your glutes to push back upward, pressing into your right heel. Touch the toes of your left foot to the bench for balance, if necessary. Return to the starting position, keeping your left foot on the bench for the next repetition. Complete 16 to 24 alternating repetitions.

BEGINNER

To help you keep your balance, use a lower bench and place it facing a wall so you can touch the wall if you need to.

INTERMEDIATE

Add a back leg lift to work both glutes. Perform the move as directed. When you step up with the first leg, lift and straighten your other leg as high as you can behind you while keeping your hips and shoulders squared. Return to the starting position. Repeat until you complete 1 set.

Minna Says
When you feel your muscles straining, your sweat running, your legs trembling . . . push harder!

ADVANCED

Add a back leg lift and knee bend. Perform the Intermediate move as described on opposite page. Before you step down, with one leg still extended behind you, bend the other knee slightly, straighten it, then return to the starting position. This move requires good balance, so do not use dumbbells until you master it.

ORIGINAL MOVE

ADVANCED MOVE

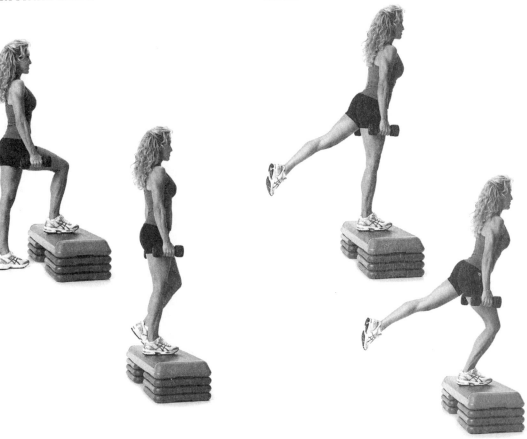

USE YOUR HEAD
The bench or step needs to be high enough to target your glutes but low enough that it doesn't stress your knees—about 15 inches high. When you step up, your knee should be at no greater than a 90-degree angle.

BREATHWORK
Exhale as you step up. Inhale as you return to the starting position. Since this move works your lungs *and* muscles, your heart rate should climb.

SUGGESTED STRETCH
Static:
Seated Forward Bend
(page 23)
and/or Modified Hurdler
(page 27)

HIP EXTENSION

*This tush-intensive move targets the glutes
without working the quadriceps, as squats and lunges do.*

SETS AND REPS

BEGINNER: 1 to 2 sets,
8 to 12 repetitions per side
INTERMEDIATE: 2 to 3 sets,
8 to 12 repetitions per side
ADVANCED: 3 sets,
8 to 12 repetitions per side

STARTING POSITION

Get down on all fours. Contract your
abdominal muscles. Keep your shoulders
and hips squared and aligned, with your
wrists directly beneath your shoulders and
your knees directly beneath your hips.
Look at the floor.

THE MOVE

Lift one leg, keeping the knee bent at a
90-degree angle, until the sole of your
foot faces the ceiling and your thigh is
parallel with the floor. Contract your
glutes on that side as hard as you can.
Lower your leg, stopping when your knee
is 2 to 3 inches from the floor. Repeat
until you complete 1 set, then switch
sides. If you're performing an odd number
of sets, switch sides halfway through
each set.

FOCUS ON FORM

♣ Distribute your weight equally among
  your hands and the knee on the floor.
  Keep your back and neck straight.
♣ Contract your abdominals throughout
  the movement.
♣ Avoid twisting or shifting your hips
  and shoulders.

AT HOME/AT THE GYM

AT HOME: Test your form. Perform the
move with a light object, such as a magazine, balanced on the small of your back.
The object should not fall. If it does,
check that your hips and shoulders are
squared and your back is straight.
AT THE GYM: Try the Butt Blaster
machine—the name says it all! Perform
the same move, but load the machine with
weighted plates.

BEGINNER

If your glutes give out before you complete
the full number of repetitions on one side,
alternate sides. If your upper body fatigues,
stay on your knees, but lower yourself
onto your forearms.

INTERMEDIATE

For an additional challenge, instead of
bending your knee, straighten your leg
and lift it up, then lower it until you can
just touch your toes to the floor. Remember to contract your abs and keep your
back straight.

ADVANCED

At the end of each set, do 1 set of 10 to 15
pulses: Pause at the top of the move, then
lift and lower your leg in the air a few
inches before bringing down your knee.

Minna Says
Often, success lies in simplicity. Simple moves like this one can do wonders.

ORIGINAL MOVE

INTERMEDIATE MOVE

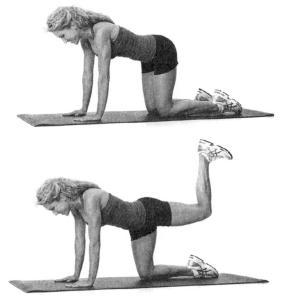

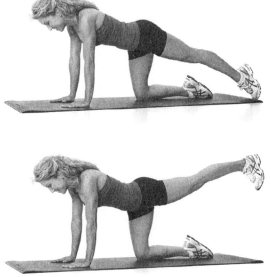

USE YOUR HEAD
At the top of the move, focus on contracting your glutes. Squeeze, squeeze, squeeze, and then, when you think you've squeezed all you can, squeeze some more. Focus, too, on keeping your spine elongated, your abdominals tight, and your hips locked.

BREATHWORK
Exhale as you lift your leg. Inhale as you lower it.

SUGGESTED STRETCH
Static:
Modified Hurdler
(page 27)

BRIDGE

This small move makes a big impact on your glutes.
It also strengthens the core muscles.

SETS AND REPS

BEGINNER: 2 sets,
10 to 15 repetitions, no weight
INTERMEDIATE: 2 to 3 sets,
10 to 15 repetitions,
8- to 12-pound dumbbell
ADVANCED: 3 sets, 10 to 15 repetitions,
8- to 12-pound dumbbell

STARTING POSITION

Lie on your back with your arms at your
sides, your knees bent, and your feet flat
on the floor about 2 feet beyond your
butt. Rest the dumbbell (if you're using
one) on your lower abdomen, holding one
end of the bar in each hand to keep it
from moving. If you're not using a dumbbell, allow your hands to rest lightly on
your abdomen.

THE MOVE

Lift your pelvis off the floor, making sure
that you don't lift the dumbbell with your
arms. Your body should make one long,
straight line from your knees to your
shoulders. Contract your glutes hard as
you lift upward, pressing into your heels.
Lower your pelvis, stopping just before
your bottom touches the floor. Repeat
until you complete 1 set.

FOCUS ON FORM

♣ Contract your abdominals throughout
the movement.
♣ Avoid excessive arching or rounding of
your back.

AT HOME/AT THE GYM

AT HOME: If you find it uncomfortable to
rest a dumbbell on your abdomen, try
using heavy books instead.
AT THE GYM: Try using a Bosu ball or
stability ball. If you use a Bosu ball, lie on
your back with your knees bent and your
feet on the ball. If you use a stability ball,
lie on your back with your legs straight
but your knees not locked, and your feet
(mainly your heels) on the ball.

BEGINNER

When you're comfortable performing the
move, add 10 to 15 pulses after each set.

INTERMEDIATE

Try this challenging variation: Cross your
right leg over your left leg at the knees,
placing your right foot on top of your left
knee so that only your left heel touches
the floor. Lift and lower your pelvis, concentrating the work into your left glutes.
Repeat until you complete 10 to 15 repetitions, then switch sides to complete 1 set.

ADVANCED

Try a one-legged version with a set of
pulses: Extend one leg straight out so that
it is aligned with the other leg's thigh. Perform 1 set and then add a set of 10 to 15
pulses. Switch sides and repeat.

ORIGINAL MOVE

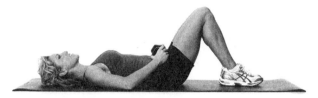

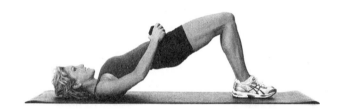

ADVANCED MOVE

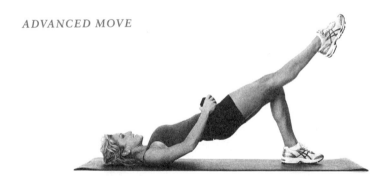

USE YOUR HEAD

Some fatigue in the hamstrings and quadriceps is normal, especially if you're a beginner. Work through it, focusing on working your glutes as best you can.

BREATHWORK

Exhale as you lift your pelvis and squeeze your glutes. Inhale as you lower your pelvis to the starting position.

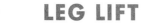
LEG LIFT

*Pack up saddlebags for good with this simple but effective move
that tones the glutes and outer thighs and improves core strength.*

SETS AND REPS

BEGINNER: 1 to 2 sets,
8 to 15 repetitions
INTERMEDIATE: 2 to 3 sets,
8 to 15 repetitions
ADVANCED: 3 sets, 10 to 15 repetitions

STARTING POSITION

Lie on your right side. Stack your hips and
shoulders. Lift yourself up onto your right
forearm. Extend your left arm in front of
and perpendicular to you, resting your
palm on the floor for balance. Your left
hand will be in front of your abdomen with
your fingertips pointing in a perpendicular
line toward your right hand. Contract your
abdominal muscles. Bend your bottom
(right) leg to about 45 degrees. Straighten
your top (left) leg and point your toes in
the direction you're facing.

THE MOVE

Without rotating your hip, lift the top
(left) leg and flex your toes slightly.
Slowly lower your top leg until just before
it touches your bottom leg. Repeat until
you complete 8 to 15 repetitions, then
switch sides, performing another 8 to 15
repetitions to complete 1 set.

FOCUS ON FORM

✤ Move slowly and with control.
✤ Keep your hips aligned with your
   shoulders. Your hips should not roll
   forward or backward.
✤ Keep your rib cage high and your
   abdominals tight.
✤ Avoiding rounding or arching your
   back.

AT HOME/AT THE GYM

AT HOME: Perform a standing side Leg
Lift. Stand with your feet hip-width apart
and bend your knees slightly. Contract
your abdominals, keeping your shoulders
and hips level and in line, and drawing
your shoulders back and down. Place your
hands on your hips. Keeping your hips
and shoulders squared, stand on your
right foot and lift your left leg sideways as
high as you can, pointing your toes forward. Return to the starting position.
AT THE GYM: Try this move on the pulley
machine. Adjust to the desired amount of
weight. Attach an ankle cuff to the low
cable of the machine, then attach the cuff
to your left ankle. Stand with your right
side next to the pulley, feet hip-width
apart, abs tight, knees slightly bent.
Slowly lift and lower your left leg until
just before the weights on the stack touch.

Minna Says
Be at peace with
your body as it
is today.

BEGINNER

If you cannot perform the move with your top leg held straight, bend your knee.

INTERMEDIATE

At the end of each set of lifts, add 8 to 15 pulses at the top of the last move.

ADVANCED

Try the modified Side Plank: Instead of keeping your hips on the floor, use your abdominals to lift them. Maintain one long, straight line from your head to your ankle. Perform 1 set of leg lifts while holding this position, then switch sides.

ORIGINAL MOVE

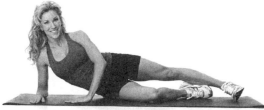

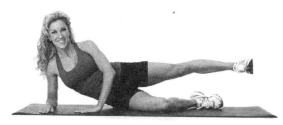

ADVANCED MOVE

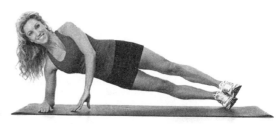

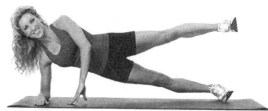

USE YOUR HEAD

Imagine that a rope attached to your ankle is gently pulling your leg up and away from your body.

BREATHWORK

Exhale as you lift your leg. Inhale as you lower it.

SUGGESTED STRETCH

Static:
Reaching Butterfly
(page 24)

KNEE/HEEL TAP

Tap your way to new heights of bootyliciousness.
This move tones the glutes and outer thighs.

SETS AND REPS

BEGINNER: 1 to 2 sets,
10 to 15 repetitions
INTERMEDIATE: 2 to 3 sets,
10 to 15 repetitions
ADVANCED: 3 sets, 10 to 15 repetitions

STARTING POSITION

Lie on your right side with your knees
bent to slightly less than 90 degrees. Stack
your shoulders and hips. Lift your rib cage
and raise yourself onto your right forearm
so that it's pointing away from your body
with your fingers flat on the floor. Contract your abdominal muscles.

THE MOVE

Raise your left leg, keeping the knee bent,
about 6 inches above your right knee.
Using your glutes, bring your left knee
down and forward until it taps the floor
slightly in front of your right knee. Your
left heel should be in the air. Using your
glutes, lower your left heel to tap the floor
in front of and just below your right knee.
Continue to alternate knee and heel taps.
Repeat until you complete 10 to 15 repetitions, then switch sides to complete 1 set.

FOCUS ON FORM

✤ Contract your abdominals throughout
the move to keep your upper body
stable.
✤ Perform this move slowly. If you rush,
you may use muscle groups other than
your glutes and upper thighs.

AT HOME/AT THE GYM

AT HOME: If you own a pair of ankle
weights, use them to perform the move.
This variation is not for beginners.
AT THE GYM: Perform a quadrupel with
Leg Abduction. Get on your hands and
knees. Raise your right leg (keeping your
knee bent) up and out to the side of your
body. Intermediate and advanced: Try to
straighten your right leg, then bend the
knee back and lower to the starting position. Beginners, just lower your bent knee.

BEGINNER

Make proper form your priority. This
move's range of motion is small but
mighty.

INTERMEDIATE

For an added challenge, hold one dumbbell alongside the thigh of your top leg,
close to your knee.

Minna Says
The burn is
temporary. A
healthy, fit body
is forever.

ADVANCED

Play with tempo. Perform the 1st set slowly, the 2nd set a little faster, and the 3rd set quickly, all while maintaining good form. Option: Add a set of lowers and lifts. Perform the move as described, then immediately lower your left

knee again and tap it in front of your right knee. Then, use your glutes to push your left leg toward the ceiling. Straighten your leg as you flex the foot, really extending through your heel as you "push." Bend your left knee and lower it again, tapping it in front of your right knee.

ORIGINAL MOVE

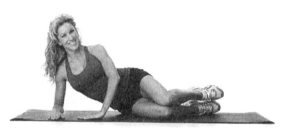

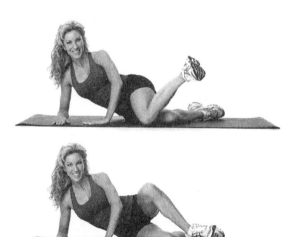

INTERMEDIATE MOVE

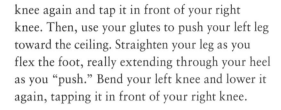

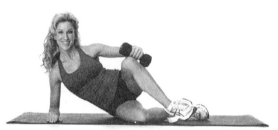

USE YOUR HEAD
Imagine that the fire in your glutes (this move *burns!*) and outer thighs is the heat of unwanted fat melting away, revealing the sculpted muscle beneath.

BREATHWORK
Exhale as you tap your knee. Inhale as you tap your heel.

SUGGESTED STRETCH
Static:
Modified Hurdler
(page 27)

LEG ABDUCTION

This move can turn a droopy backside into what's known as a "high-water booty." It lifts and firms the glutes, tones the outer thighs, and improves core strength.

SETS AND REPS

BEGINNER: 1 to 2 sets,
8 to 12 repetitions per leg
INTERMEDIATE: 2 to 3 sets,
8 to 12 repetitions per leg
ADVANCED: 3 sets,
8 to 12 repetitions per leg

STARTING POSITION

Get down on all fours, placing your hands directly beneath your shoulders and your knees directly beneath your hips. Contract your abdominal muscles and square your hips and shoulders. Keeping your head aligned with your spine, look at the floor.

THE MOVE

Lift your left leg upward and outward, keeping your knee bent, until your thigh is parallel with the floor. Return to the starting position. Repeat until you complete 8 to 12 repetitions, then switch sides to complete 1 set.

FOCUS ON FORM

- ❖ Distribute your weight equally among your hands and the knee on the floor.
- ❖ Avoid leaning to the side as you lift.
- ❖ Contract your abdominals throughout the move to maintain your balance and protect your lower back.

AT HOME/AT THE GYM

AT HOME: Try a standing side leg kick. Stand with your feet hip-width apart. Contract your abdominals. Clench your fists and lift your bent arms in front of your face and chest, as if you were defending yourself against a punch. Lift your left leg, bend your left knee, and immediately extend it straight to the side. Flexing your heel, kick to the side as if you were going to kick a punching bag with your heel. Return to the starting position. Repeat to complete 8 to 12 repetitions, then switch sides to complete 1 set.

AT THE GYM: Try this move on the outer thigh abductor machine. (Ask a trainer to assist you, if necessary.) When you are comfortable with the machine and the move, lean forward slightly on the seat to more precisely target your glutes.

BEGINNER

If the starting position tires you out, perform the move while lying on your side with your knees bent in front of you. Start with your legs stacked on top of each other and your feet together. Lift your top leg until it is almost perpendicular to the floor, then return to the starting position. Repeat to complete 8 to 12 repetitions, then switch sides to complete 1 set.

Minna Says
Give each workout your all. Consistent effort brings consistent results.

INTERMEDIATE

Add a straight leg extension: At the top of the move, straighten and extend your left (top) leg while flexing your foot and keeping your toes pointing toward the floor. Lengthen your leg through your heel. Then return to the starting position. Repeat to complete 8 to 12 repetitions, then switch sides to complete 1 set.

ADVANCED

From the starting position, straighten your left leg and swing it around so that it extends to the side. Lift it until it is parallel with the floor, then lower it to a point just before your foot touches the floor. Repeat to complete 8 to 12 repetitions, then switch sides to complete 1 set.

ORIGINAL MOVE

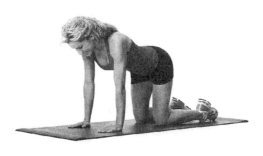

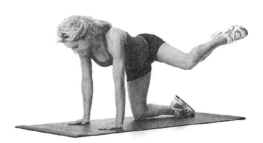

ADVANCED MOVE

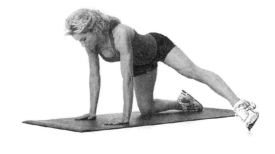

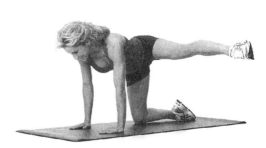

USE YOUR HEAD

Think of a table with a hanging leaf. The table—your body—remains solid and immovable. The leaf—the leg you're lifting—rises to the height of the table.

BREATHWORK

Exhale as you lift your leg. Inhale as you lower it.

SUGGESTED STRETCH

Static:
Modified Hurdler
(page 27)

♣

STATIONARY LUNGE

Think of this move as a facelift for your bottom. It firms, lifts, and tightens the glutes and tones the quadriceps.

SETS AND REPS

BEGINNER: 1 to 2 sets,
8 to 12 repetitions per leg,
no weight or 5- to 8-pound dumbbells
INTERMEDIATE: 2 to 3 sets,
8 to 12 repetitions per leg,
8- to 12-pound dumbbells
ADVANCED: 3 sets,
8 to 12 repetitions per leg,
12- to 25-pound dumbbells

STARTING POSITION

Stand with your feet hip-width apart, holding dumbbells at your sides with your palms facing inward. Contract your abdominal muscles, square your shoulders and hips, and draw your shoulders back and down. Take a giant step forward with your left leg; lift the heel of your right foot, but leave the foot at that location. Distribute your weight evenly between both feet.

THE MOVE

Bend your knees and lower your body until your front (left) thigh is parallel with the floor. Pressing your weight into your left heel, use your glutes to return to the starting position. Repeat until you complete 8 to 12 repetitions, then switch legs to complete 1 set. If you're performing an odd number of sets, switch legs halfway through each set.

> **Minna Says**
> Music can be just as motivating as a personal trainer. Put on your favorite tunes, get into the zone, and go for it.

FOCUS ON FORM

♣ Contract your abdominals throughout the move to support your lower back.
♣ To help you maintain your balance, keep your hips and shoulders squared throughout the move.
♣ Bend your front knee to 90 degrees only, and keep it directly over your ankle. Allowing your knee to creep past your toes stresses the joint.
♣ Really press into your front heel as you rise to target the glute.

AT HOME/AT THE GYM

AT HOME: Alternate the move with the Plié Squat (see page 192). Perform one Stationary Lunge with your right leg forward. Then, pivot on your left leg and do a quarter-turn into a Plié Squat. Perform one Plié Squat, resting the dumbbells on your thighs, then pivot again for another quarter-turn, so that your left leg is forward and your right leg is back. Perform another Stationary Lunge. Continue to alternate the Stationary Lunge with the Plié Squat, making quarter-turns between the moves. Repeat until you complete 1 set of 16 to 24 alternating lunges.

AT THE GYM: Use the Smith Machine. Adjust the bar on the machine so that it is below shoulder level. Place a flat bench 12 to 18 inches behind the path of the bar. With the bar across your shoulders, bend your back leg and rest your toes on the bench. Test the spacing to make sure it's right—when you lower yourself, the knee of the front leg should be directly over your foot. Perform the move. Complete 8 to 12 repetitions, then switch sides. This variation is for advanced readers only.

BEGINNER
Until you familiarize yourself with this exercise, hold on to the back of a chair for added balance.

INTERMEDIATE
At the bottom of the movement, hold for a count of three before rising. This should create some fire!

ADVANCED
After completing each set, immediately perform the T Pose (page 200). Hold the T Pose for 10 to 30 seconds, then switch legs.

ORIGINAL MOVE

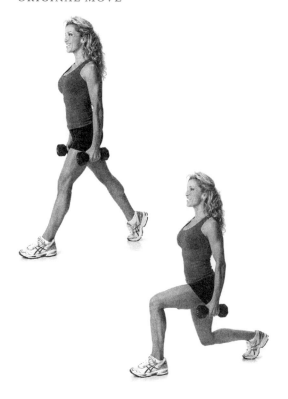

ADVANCED MOVE

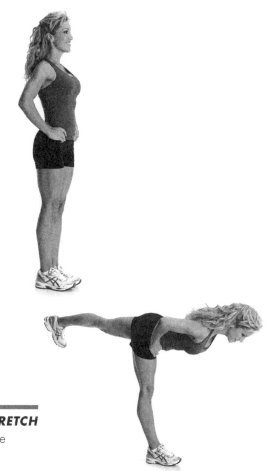

USE YOUR HEAD
Think of your dumbbells as two brimming pails of water. The goal is to lower and lift yourself so smoothly, gracefully, and linearly that not a drop is spilled.

SUGGESTED STRETCH
Kneeling Lunge
(page 25)

8

BOY SHORTS BOTTOM
SKILLED

If you've mastered the Novice moves or worked out with weights prior to starting my program, these lower body exercises are for you. They demand more strength and balance than the Novice moves and really zero in on your thighs, hips, and glutes. Again, you'll see quicker, more dramatic results if you team them with a sensible eating plan and at least 30 minutes of aerobic exercise on most or all days of the week. If you are working out at home, you'll need a Bosu ball and/or a stability ball if you wish to try the variations in the "At the Gym" sections.

FEATURED EXERCISES:
♣ALTERNATING REVERSE LUNGE
♣CURTSY LUNGE
♣FROGGY DOUBLE-LEG LIFT
♣SIDE LUNGE
♣PLIÉ SQUAT
♣STANDING HIP EXTENSION

ALTERNATING REVERSE LUNGE

This move will prep your bottom for the bitsiest pair of boy shorts.
It builds and sculpts the glutes, tones the quadriceps, and improves balance.

SETS AND REPS

BEGINNER: 1 to 2 sets,
16 to 24 alternating repetitions,
no weight or 5-pound dumbbells
INTERMEDIATE: 2 to 3 sets,
16 to 24 alternating repetitions,
8- to 15-pound dumbbells
ADVANCED: 3 sets,
16 to 24 alternating repetitions,
12- to 25-pound dumbbells

STARTING POSITION

Stand with your feet together. Hold the dumbbells at your sides, palms facing inward. Contract your abdominal muscles, square your shoulders and hips, and draw your shoulders back and down.

THE MOVE

Take a giant step backward with your left foot, lowering your left knee toward the floor as you bend your right knee to 90 degrees. Keep your hips squared and facing forward. Lower yourself until your right thigh is parallel with the floor and your left knee is 1 to 2 inches from the floor. Distribute your weight evenly between both feet. Return to the starting position, pressing your weight into the heel of your right foot as you do so. Repeat, this time stepping backward with your right foot. Alternate sides until you complete 1 set.

Minna Says
Never say "I can't."
Instead, say "I'll try."
The doors of
possibility will
fly open.

FOCUS ON FORM

❖ Contract your abdominals throughout the move to protect your lower back.
❖ Keep your front knee directly over your ankle to protect your knees.
❖ If you feel the burn in the front of your thighs, try to kindle that "burn" in your bottom. Press into the heel of your front leg to make your glutes work harder than your quads.

AT HOME/AT THE GYM

AT HOME: Beginners, try a few practice lunges. Place a towel or other marker on the floor so you know where your back foot should land. Intermediate and advanced readers, put down your dumbbells and add a split-leg jump. At the bottom of the move (when you are in the lunge, with your right leg forward and your left leg back), jump into the air and scissor your legs so that their positions are reversed when you land. Immediately bend your knees and lower yourself into the lunge. Repeat until you complete 1 set of 12 to 20 alternating repetitions.

AT THE GYM: Try this move on the Smith Machine. Place the desired amount of weight on the machine. If your gym has a shoulder pad, pop it into place around the bar for added comfort. With your back to the machine, stand about 12 inches in front of it and place the bar across your shoulders. Shift the bar backward to unlock the weight. Perform the move.

BEGINNER

If it's tough to keep your balance, steady yourself by touching the back of a chair or the wall.

INTERMEDIATE

Add a leg raise to work both legs' glutes, rather than just the glutes of your front leg: Perform the move. As you return to the starting position, lift your back leg as high as you can while maintaining proper form. If you feel the move in your lower back, you are lifting your leg too high.

ADVANCED

Add a T Pose (see page 200). Perform the move. As you return to the starting position, lift your back leg and simultaneously lower your torso so that your body forms a T shape. Hold for 2 to 3 seconds, return to the starting position, and switch sides.

ORIGINAL MOVE

INTERMEDIATE MOVE

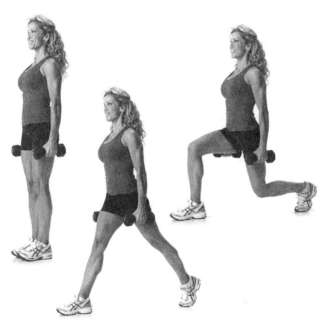

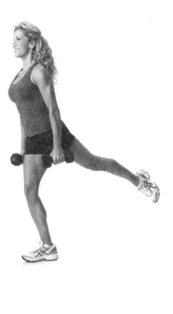

USE YOUR HEAD

As you lower yourself into the lunge, focus on contracting the glutes of your front leg. As you return to the starting position, squeeze them as hard as you can.

BREATHWORK

Inhale as you lower yourself into the lunge. Exhale as you return to the starting position.

SUGGESTED STRETCH

Moving Flexibility:
Split Leg
(page 34)

CURTSY LUNGE

This move can buff up a less-than-perky bum by shaping and toning the glutes.

SETS AND REPS

BEGINNER: 1 to 2 sets, 8 to 12 repetitions, no weight at first, progressing to 5- to 8-pound dumbbells
INTERMEDIATE: 2 to 3 sets, 8 to 12 repetitions, 8- to 12-pound dumbbells
ADVANCED: 3 sets, 8 to 12 repetitions, 12- to 25-pound dumbbells

STARTING POSITION

Holding the dumbbells at your sides with your palms facing inward, stand with your feet together. Contract your abdominal muscles and keep your shoulders and hips squared and aligned. Draw your shoulders back and down.

THE MOVE

Keeping the dumbbells at your sides, take a giant step backward and diagonally with your right foot, crossing your right leg behind your left and bending your knees, as if you were dropping into a curtsy. Keep your torso upright. Push through your heels to return to the starting position. Repeat until you complete 8 to 12 repetitions, then switch sides to complete 1 set.

Minna Says
Positive thoughts lead to positive results.

FOCUS ON FORM

❦ Contract your abdominals throughout the move to support your lower back.
❦ Position your front knee directly over your foot.

AT HOME/AT THE GYM

AT HOME: Assume the starting position. Instead of lunging backward, take a giant diagonal step forward, crossing your midline by 12 inches. (Imagine a line drawn straight down the middle of your body, from your head to your feet. That line is your midline.)
AT THE GYM: Try this move on the leg press machine. Add the desired amount of weight to the machine. Sit down and place one foot on the flat surface. Rotate your foot inward 2 to 3 inches. Release the safety latch and slowly lower the weight by bringing your knee toward your chest, keeping your knee in line with your toes. Repeat until you complete 8 to 12 repetitions, then switch legs to complete 1 set.

BEGINNER

If you need to, hold on to the wall or the back of a sturdy chair for balance. Also, if this move fatigues your lower back, alternate legs for 1 set.

INTERMEDIATE

Perform the move. As you return to the starting position, keep your weight on your working (left) leg and simply tap the toes of your right foot on the floor for balance.

ADVANCED

As you perform the move, lower your torso as you would if you were reaching for a pen you had dropped. Then return to the starting position. This variation is not for beginners or for those who have discomfort in or an injury of the lower back.

ORIGINAL MOVE

ADVANCED MOVE

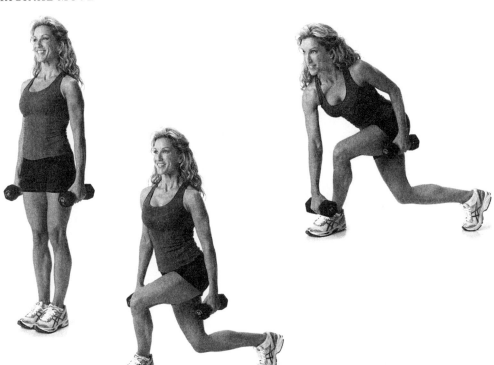

USE YOUR HEAD
You should feel this move in your glutes only. Think of your torso, arms, and legs as the movable parts of a handheld puppet and your glutes as the hand directing those moves.

BREATHWORK
Inhale as you lower yourself into the lunge. Exhale as you return to the starting position.

SUGGESTED STRETCH
Static:
Spinal Twist
(page 31)
Moving Flexibility:
Walking Quadriceps
(page 40)

FROGGY DOUBLE-LEG LIFT

The froggy may look funny, but it will seriously improve your "rear view."
This move tones the glutes and hamstrings.

SETS AND REPS

BEGINNER: 1 to 2 sets,
10 to 15 repetitions
INTERMEDIATE: 2 to 3 sets,
10 to 15 repetitions
ADVANCED: 3 sets, 10 to 15 repetitions

STARTING POSITION

Lie on your belly on the floor with your legs flat on the floor and your knees bent to 90 degrees and hip-width apart. (Yes, you look like a frog.) Touch your heels together and turn your feet so your toes point outward. Cross your forearms in front of you and rest your forehead on them. Contract your abdominal muscles.

THE MOVE

Using your glutes, lift your thighs as far off the floor as you can *without* using the muscles in your lower back. Contract your glutes hard for 2 to 3 seconds, then return to the starting position. Repeat until you complete 1 set.

FOCUS ON FORM

♣ Avoid contracting your hamstrings or lower back muscles to lift your legs.
♣ Squeeze, squeeze, squeeze those glutes—it's not about how high you lift but how hard you squeeze.
♣ Every few repetitions, check your shoulders. If they are rising toward your ears, you are lifting your legs too high.

BEGINNER

If you can't lift your thighs off the floor, keep trying! Until then, just squeeze your glutes as hard as you can.

INTERMEDIATE

Perform the move as directed, but before lowering your thighs, separate your heels and extend your legs until they are almost straight. Then bend your knees, bring your heels together, and lower your thighs.

ADVANCED

After performing 1 set of the move, add 1 set of pulses and/or straight-leg heel taps. Heel taps: After the last repetition of a set, straighten your legs and space your feet, with your toes turned outward, 12 inches apart. Use your glutes to lift your legs off the floor. Then, squeezing your glutes, bring your heels back together with a tap. Perform 10 to 15 repetitions.

ORIGINAL MOVE

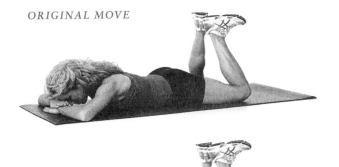

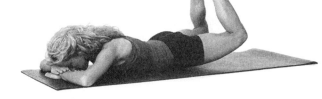

ADVANCED MOVE

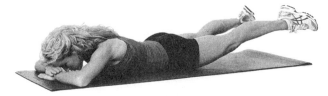

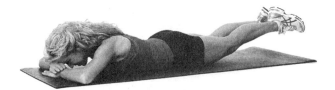

USE YOUR HEAD

If you feel this move in your lower back, focus on contracting *only* your glutes as you relax the muscles of your lower back.

BREATHWORK

Exhale as you lift your legs. Inhale as you lower them.

SUGGESTED STRETCH

Static:
Reaching Butterfly
(page 24)

SIDE LUNGE

Lunge your way to a perfectly proportioned lower body. This move shapes the glutes and outer thighs, strengthens the quadriceps and hamstrings, and improves core strength and balance.

SETS AND REPS

BEGINNER: 1 to 2 sets, 8 to 12 repetitions, no weight at first, then 5- to 8-pound dumbbells

INTERMEDIATE: 2 to 3 sets, 8 to 12 repetitions, 8- to 12-pound dumbbells

ADVANCED: 3 sets, 8 to 12 repetitions, 12- to 25-pound dumbbells

STARTING POSITION

Holding the dumbbells at your sides with your palms facing inward, stand with your feet together. Contract your abdominal muscles and draw your shoulders back and down.

THE MOVE

Keeping your left leg straight, lift your right foot, bend your right knee, and take a large step to the side with your right foot. Keep your toes pointing forward and your knee directly over your ankle. Lower yourself until your right thigh is parallel with the floor. Keep your torso upright and both feet facing forward. Using your glutes, return to the starting position. Repeat until you complete 8 to 12 repetitions, then switch sides to complete 1 set.

Minna Says
Strive for proper form. It's the foundation of a successful strength-training program and the key to staying injury-free.

FOCUS ON FORM

* Contract your abdominals throughout the move to protect your lower back.
* Keep your chest lifted as you lower into the move.
* Keep your bent knee directly over your ankle.

AT HOME/AT THE GYM

AT HOME: Perform the move without dumbbells. Raise your arms over your head and curve them as though you are hugging a beach ball. As you lunge to the right, twist your torso to the right slightly and bring your arms down, across, and past your right knee, as if you were placing the ball on the floor. Then, pick up your imaginary ball and sweep your arms over your head.

AT THE GYM: To work your upper body as well as down below, use a medicine ball. Assume the starting position, holding the ball to your chest. As you step into the lunge, lower the ball toward the floor with your arms. As you stand up, press the ball over your head. Keep your torso upright throughout the move.

BEGINNER

If you are not using weights, place your hands on your hips for balance as you perform the move. Also, if your back gets tired, alternate sides.

INTERMEDIATE

As you return to the starting position, instead of placing your working foot back on the floor, bend your knee and lift your foot 2 to 12 inches off the floor. If need be, quickly tap your toes to the floor for balance.

ORIGINAL MOVE

ADVANCED

Add a front lunge. Perform the move as directed. As you return to the starting position, take a large step forward with the same leg, moving into a forward lunge. Keep your knee directly over your toes, bending it until your thigh is parallel with the floor. Return to the starting position.

ADVANCED MOVE

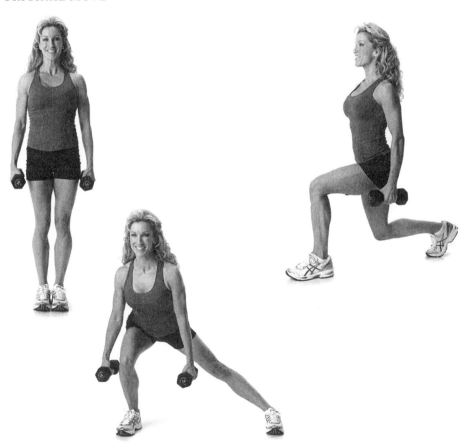

USE YOUR HEAD

As you lower yourself into the move, push your hips backward slightly, as if you were about to sit in a chair.

BREATHWORK

Inhale as you lower yourself into the lunge. Exhale as you return to the starting position.

SUGGESTED STRETCH
Static:
Modified Hurdler
(page 27)

PLIÉ SQUAT

This classic ballet move helps give ballerinas their strong, shapely lower bodies. It builds and sculpts the glutes, inner thighs, and quadriceps.

SETS AND REPS

BEGINNER: 1 to 2 sets,
8 to 12 repetitions,
no weight or 5- to 8-pound dumbbell
INTERMEDIATE: 2 to 3 sets,
8 to 12 repetitions,
8- to 15-pound dumbbell
ADVANCED: 3 sets, 8 to 12 repetitions,
15- to 25-pound dumbbell

STARTING POSITION

Stand with your feet slightly wider than shoulder-width apart, holding the dumbbell vertically in front of you with both hands, with your palms faceup, cupping the upper end of the weight. Turn your feet so that your toes point outward and align your knees in the same direction as your toes. Contract your abdominals, square your shoulders and hips, and draw your shoulders back and down.

THE MOVE

Keeping your torso upright and your knees directly over your toes, slowly lower your body until your thighs are parallel with the floor. Use your glutes to slowly rise and return to the starting position.

FOCUS ON FORM

❖ Keep your feet slightly wider than shoulder-width apart.
❖ Keep your upper body erect. Leaning forward places stress on your lower back.
❖ Point your knees in the same direction as your toes.
❖ Use your glutes throughout the move. Contract them to hold the turned-outward position of your legs; squeeze them as you lower and lift.

BEGINNER

If you cannot rotate your legs outward so that your knees follow the direction of your toes, focus on contracting your glutes to open your legs more. This tip, and the stretch suggested on the opposite page, will help improve your flexibility.

INTERMEDIATE

Add a heel lift. Perform the move, but lift your heels off the floor (it's harder than you might think). Or lift your heels as you lower into the squat, rise with your heels still lifted, and then lower them when you return to the starting position.

ADVANCED

After each set of Plié Squats, perform a set of plyometric Plié Squats—the same move, only airborne. After you complete the last repetition of a set, put down your dumbbell and immediately spring into the air, legs apart. When you land, immediately bend your knees and lower yourself into the plié for another jump. Repeat until you complete 1 set (8 to 12 repetitions).

ORIGINAL MOVE

ADVANCED MOVE

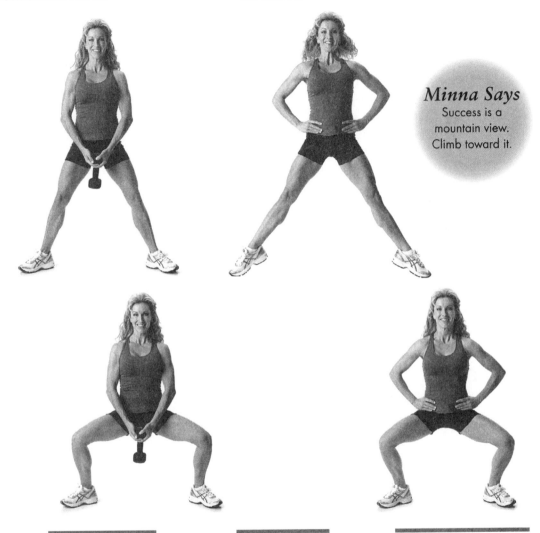

Minna Says
Success is a
mountain view.
Climb toward it.

USE YOUR HEAD
As you perform this move, imagine
that you have the effortless grace of
a ballet dancer. Do a total body
mental scan: Your chin and chest
should be lifted, your shoulders
should be relaxed and down, your
abs should be contracted, and your
legs should be rotated outward.

BREATHWORK
Inhale as you lower yourself into
the move. Exhale as you return to
the starting position.

SUGGESTED STRETCH
Static:
Reaching Butterfly
(page 24)

STANDING HIP EXTENSION

This move will have you slipping into boy shorts in no time. It sculpts the glutes, strengthens the hamstrings and erector spinae muscles (which run along the spine), and improves balance.

SETS AND REPS

BEGINNER: 1 to 2 sets,
8 to 12 repetitions per leg
INTERMEDIATE: 2 to 3 sets,
8 to 12 repetitions per leg
ADVANCED: 3 sets,
8 to 12 repetitions per leg

STARTING POSITION

Stand with your feet together and your hands on your hips. Bend your knees slightly, square your hips and shoulders, and draw your shoulders back and down. Contract your abdominal muscles.

THE MOVE

Using your glutes, lift your left leg behind your body, pointing your toes at the floor and keeping your torso upright. Lift your leg as high as you can, using only your glutes and maintaining proper form. Lower your leg to the starting position. Repeat until you complete 8 to 12 repetitions, then switch legs to complete 1 set. If you are performing an odd number of sets, switch legs halfway through each set.

FOCUS ON FORM

✤ Focus not on how high you lift your leg but on how hard you squeeze your glutes.
✤ Arching your back is not necessary. Use only your glutes.
✤ Contract your abdominals throughout the move to help you balance.

AT HOME/AT THE GYM

AT HOME: Beginners, if you need to, hold the back of a chair for balance. Intermediate and advanced readers, try the donkey kick jump. Perform the move as described, but continuously hop from foot to foot, kicking your leg back behind you as your arms mimic the motion of jumping rope. Perform 20 to 30 alternating jumps.

AT THE GYM: Perform the move on the cable machine. Add the desired amount of weight. Buckle the cuff onto your right ankle, then attach it to the lower cable. Face the machine, holding the bar for balance. Perform 8 to 12 repetitions with your right leg, then switch legs.

BEGINNER

Do the quadruped leg lift. Get down on all fours with your hands positioned beneath your shoulders and your knees beneath your hips. Contract your abdominals. Extend your right leg straight back, then lift it until it is parallel with the floor. Keeping the leg straight, lower it until just before your toes touch the floor, then lift it again.

Minna Says
Never say never.
Instead, say,
"Next time."

INTERMEDIATE

Perform the move as directed, but do not return to the starting position. Instead, lower your leg until just before your toes touch the floor. Repeat until you complete 8 to 12 repetitions, then switch sides to complete 1 set.

ADVANCED

After performing 1 set of the move with your left leg, return to the starting position and lift your right heel, keeping your toes on the floor for balance. Push your hips backward and lower yourself into a One-Legged Squat on your left leg. Return to the starting position. Repeat until you complete 8 to 12 repetitions, then switch sides to complete 1 set.

ORIGINAL MOVE

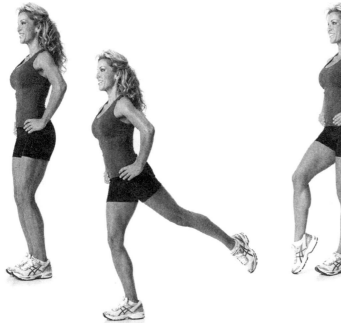

ADVANCED MOVE

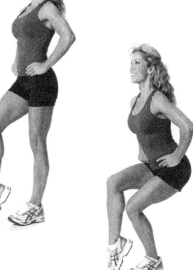

USE YOUR HEAD

Picture a retractable string attaching your glutes to your lifting foot. Each time you contract your glutes, the contraction pulls the string, lifting your leg.

SUGGESTED STRETCH
Static:
Modified Hurdler
(page 27)

9

BOY SHORTS BOTTOM
MASTER

Think you can't do any more to lift your fanny, firm your thighs, and trim your hips? You ain't seen nothing yet. These moves are for you if you've mastered the Skilled exercises or worked out with weights prior to starting my program. They provide the ultimate lower body challenge, requiring considerable strength, balance, and flexibility. As an advanced reader, you already know that you should combine these moves with a healthy diet and regular cardio for optimal results. If you are working out at home, you'll need a Bosu ball and/or a stability ball to perform the variations in the "At the Gym" sections.

FEATURED EXERCISES:

♣DEAD LIFT

♣T POSE

♣SPLIT-LEG LUNGE

♣ONE-LEGGED SQUAT

♣REVERSE PLANK WITH LEG LIFT

♣WALKING LUNGE

DEAD LIFT

This move is one of the best booty-shapers there is.
It sculpts the glutes and strengthens the hamstrings.

SETS AND REPS

BEGINNER: 1 to 2 sets,
8 to 12 repetitions, 5-pound dumbbells
INTERMEDIATE: 2 to 3 sets,
8 to 12 repetitions,
8- to 15-pound dumbbells
ADVANCED: 3 sets, 8 to 12 repetitions,
12- to 25-pound dumbbells.
Use less weight for the first set until you
warm up, then increase the weight
for sets 2 and 3.

STARTING POSITION

Stand with your feet together, holding the
dumbbells horizontally in front of your
thighs with your palms facing toward you.
Contract the muscles of your abdomen
and your lower back. Draw your shoulders back and down.

THE MOVE

Bend forward at the hips, caving your
back slightly to lift your tailbone, and
lower your torso as far as you can without
having to bend your knees (you should be
at least parallel with the floor). Hold the
dumbbells close to your shins and directly
under your shoulders. Pause when you feel
a stretch in your hamstrings. Pushing up
through your heels, return to
the starting position.
Squeeze those glutes hard!

Minna Says
An ounce of action
means more than
a ton of words.

FOCUS ON FORM

✤ While performing the move, keep your
head up and your eyes directed in front
of you.
✤ Position your ankles directly under
your knees and your knees directly
under your hips.
✤ Throughout the move, contract your
abs and lift your tailbone.

AT HOME/AT THE GYM

AT HOME: If you are very flexible, consider trying this move while standing on
the bottom step of a staircase to extend
the length of your stretch. This variation
is not for beginners.
AT THE GYM: Try this move with a Bosu
ball or core board. At first, use lighter
dumbbells than you usually do, because
your core muscles will have to work
harder to stabilize your body. Work toward executing this move as fluidly as
possible.

BEGINNER

Lower your torso only until it is parallel
with the floor. Also, keep your knees
slightly bent throughout the move.

INTERMEDIATE

Try to lower your torso closer to the floor
without bending your knees.

ADVANCED

Once you master the basic move, try the challenging one-legged version. Holding your dumbbells in front of your thighs, place one leg 2 to 3 feet behind the other with only your toes touching the floor. Bend the front knee slightly.

Keeping your shoulders back, your abs tight, and your back straight, lower the dumbbells toward the floor, bending only at the hips. Lower your torso until it is almost parallel with the floor. Push up through your heel to return to the starting position.

ORIGINAL MOVE

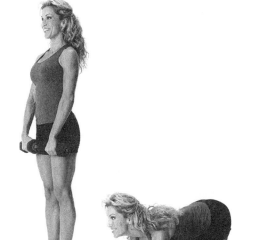

ADVANCED MOVE

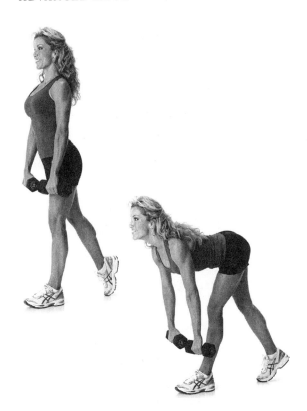

USE YOUR HEAD

Think of your body as being one long, unbroken line with no movable parts except for your hips.

BREATHWORK

Inhale as you lower your torso. Exhale as you return to the starting position.

SUGGESTED STRETCH

Static:
Seated Forward Bend
(page 23)

T POSE

This classic yoga pose is also an intense butt-blaster. It firms the glutes, strengthens the hamstrings and core, and improves balance and coordination.

SETS AND REPS

BEGINNER: 1 to 2 sets;
hold for 5 to 10 seconds
INTERMEDIATE: 2 to 3 sets;
hold for 5 to 15 seconds
ADVANCED: 3 sets;
hold for 10 to 30 seconds

STARTING POSITION

Stand with your feet together, hands on your hips. Contract your abdominal muscles and square and align your shoulders and hips.

THE MOVE

Bend forward at the hips to lower your torso as you simultaneously lift your left leg behind you until your torso and leg are parallel with the floor and your body makes one long line from your head to your left heel. If you can't fully extend your right knee, bend it slightly. Hold for the amount of time recommended for your fitness level, breathing deeply and rhythmically through your nose. Return to the starting position, then switch sides and repeat to complete 1 set.

FOCUS ON FORM

✤ Focus your gaze on an object on the floor directly below where your head will be to keep your head and neck aligned.
✤ Contract your leg muscles, glutes, abs, and lower back muscles.
✤ For balance, contract your glutes hard and keep your foot flat on the floor.
✤ Breathe deeply.

AT HOME/AT THE GYM

AT HOME: Beginners, to perform the full T Pose, hold the back of a sturdy chair for balance. Intermediate and advanced readers, perform the move as described below.
AT THE GYM: Perform this move on a Bosu ball or core board. This variation is not for beginners.

BEGINNER

Until you master form and balance, allow the toes of your back leg to touch the floor and lower your torso to only a 45-degree angle. Lift your toes from the floor when you can hold the Beginner position for 5 seconds. Once your balance improves, work toward reaching the full T Pose.

INTERMEDIATE

Extend your arms straight out to the sides, lining them up with your shoulders.

ADVANCED

Perform knee bends on your standing leg: Place your hands on your hips or extend your arms out to the sides for balance. When your torso is bent forward and is parallel with the floor, lower yourself 2 to 6 inches. Repeat until you complete 5 to 10 knee bends. Switch sides and complete 5 to 10 more to finish 1 set.

ORIGINAL MOVE

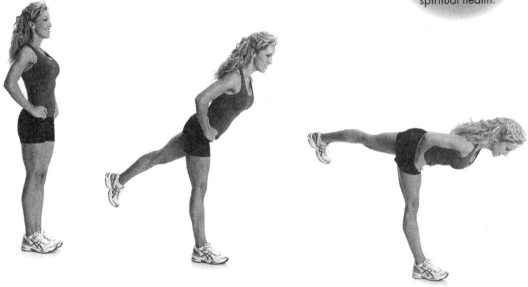

ADVANCED MOVE

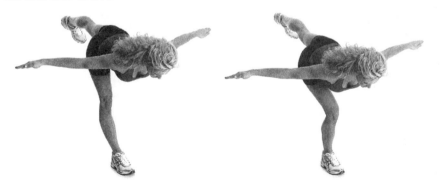

USE YOUR HEAD
To keep your balance and ease muscle fatigue, visualize the leg you're standing on as a steel bar—strong, immobile, unbreakable.

BREATHWORK
Be sure to keep breathing as you hold this pose.

SUGGESTED STRETCH
Moving Flexibility:
Lying Leg Split
(page 36)
Perform 1 set after each T Pose.

SPLIT-LEG LUNGE

This move works the glutes and hamstrings hard, toning the glutes, increasing flexibility in the hamstrings, and shaping the quadriceps. Your reward: a bodacious backside.

SETS AND REPS

BEGINNER: 1 to 2 sets,
8 to 12 repetitions, no weight
INTERMEDIATE: 2 to 3 sets,
8 to 12 repetitions,
3- to 8-pound dumbbells
ADVANCED: 3 sets,
8 to 12 repetitions,
5- to 15-pound dumbbells

STARTING POSITION

Stand with your feet hip-width apart with your hands on your hips (if not using dumbbells) or holding the dumbbells at your sides with your palms turned inward. Contract your abdominal muscles, stack your hips and shoulders, and draw your shoulders back and down. Take a large step backward with your left foot so that your feet are 3 to 4 feet apart. Distribute your weight equally between both feet. Bending at the hips, lower your torso until it is parallel or almost parallel with the floor. Keep your legs straight (if necessary, bend your knees slightly).

THE MOVE

From the starting position, bend both knees, lowering yourself until your right thigh is parallel with the floor. Use your glutes to push your hips back up, lifting your tailbone toward the ceiling. You will feel an added stretch in your hamstrings. Return to the starting position. Repeat until you complete 8 to 12 repetitions, then switch sides to complete 1 set.

FOCUS ON FORM

✤ Contract your abdominal muscles throughout the move.
✤ When you straighten your legs and push your hips back up, press into your forward heel to increase the glutes' workload.
✤ Keep your gaze leveled in front of you. Looking at the floor can make your neck stiff.

AT HOME/AT THE GYM

AT HOME: Perform a moving warrior. Stand with your feet hip-width apart, hands on your hips, abs tight, hips and shoulders squared. Take a large step backward with your left foot, keeping your left leg straight but bending your right knee. Turn your back (left) foot slightly outward. Keep your forward (right) foot pointing forward. Distribute your weight evenly between your feet. Inhale deeply and lower your torso until it is almost parallel with the floor. Use your glutes and back muscles to lift your torso to the starting position, exhaling as you do so. Complete 5 to 10 repetitions on each side.
AT THE GYM: Try this move on a Bosu ball (without dumbbells at first), placing your front leg on the ball. This variation is not for beginners.

BEGINNER

Hold on to the back of a sturdy chair or a wall for balance.

INTERMEDIATE

Work toward mastering the technique and improving your hamstrings' flexibility. With every repetition, try to lift your tailbone higher toward the ceiling.

ORIGINAL MOVE

ADVANCED

After completing each set of lunges, move immediately into the T Pose (see page 200). Hold for 10 to 30 seconds, breathing deeply.

ADVANCED MOVE

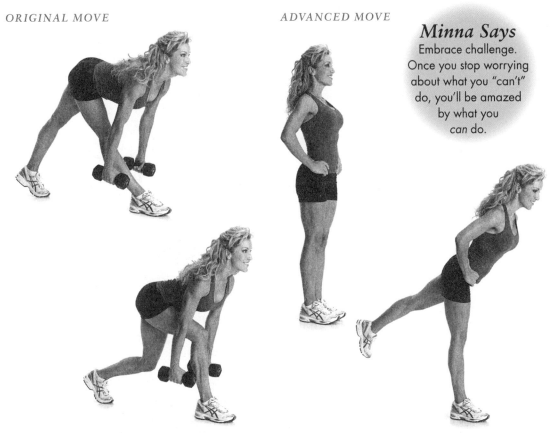

Minna Says
Embrace challenge. Once you stop worrying about what you "can't" do, you'll be amazed by what you *can* do.

USE YOUR HEAD
Think of your hamstrings as the legs of a wrinkled pair of pants. Visualize an iron moving slowly up the fabric, smoothing and lengthening the fibers.

BREATHWORK
Inhale as you bend your knee and lower your thigh. Exhale as you return to the starting position.

SUGGESTED STRETCH
Moving Flexibility:
Lying Leg Split
(page 36)

ONE-LEGGED SQUAT

This move will allow you to wear anything—or nothing at all—with pride.
It shapes and tones the glutes and improves balance and coordination.

SETS AND REPS

BEGINNER: 1 to 2 sets,
8 to 12 repetitions per leg, no weight
or 1- to 8-pound dumbbells
INTERMEDIATE: 2 to 3 sets,
8 to 12 repetitions per leg,
5- to 12-pound dumbbells
ADVANCED: 3 sets,
8 to 12 repetitions per leg,
10- to 20-pound dumbbells

STARTING POSITION

Hold the dumbbells at your sides, palms facing inward. (If you're not using dumbbells, place your hands on your hips.) Stand with your feet hip-width apart, abdominal muscles contracted, hips and shoulders squared, and shoulders drawn back and down. Shift your weight onto your left foot. Lift your right heel, bending your knee slightly, and position your right foot so that your toes are 6 to 12 inches forward of the toes of your left foot. Your feet should still be hip-width apart.

THE MOVE

Bend your left knee and push your hips backward and down as if you were going to sit in a chair. Keep your weight on your left foot, especially in the heel. Pressing into your left heel, use your glutes to return to the starting position. Repeat until you complete 8 to 12 repetitions, then switch sides to complete 1 set.

FOCUS ON FORM

✤ It's okay if you can't lower your body as far as you can when you are executing the regular Squat. Lower yourself as much as you can while still maintaining proper form.
✤ Really push your hips backward—this motion places the workload on the glutes.
✤ Contract your abdominals throughout the move to support your lower back and to assist with balance.
✤ Keep your chest lifted by squeezing your shoulder blades together.

AT HOME/AT THE GYM

AT HOME: To make it easier for your back and quads, try a one-legged Bridge. Lie on your back with your knees bent and your feet flat on floor and about 12 inches beyond your butt. Lift and straighten your left leg so it is over your left hip. Press into your right heel and use your glutes to lift your pelvis off the floor. Squeeze your right glute hard, then lower your leg until it almost touches the floor. Perform 8 to 12 repetitions on each side to complete 1 set.
AT THE GYM: Try a one-legged leg press. Ask a trainer to help you adjust the leg press machine for your height. Add the desired amount of weight. Place your right foot at the center of the foot pad, keeping your left leg relaxed and down. Release the safety brake. Bend your right knee and lower the weight by bringing your right knee toward your chest. Push the weight back up by pressing into your right heel.

BEGINNER

For added balance and stability, hold on to the back of a chair or the wall, and/or shift some of your weight to your nonworking leg.

INTERMEDIATE

To challenge your balance, try to lift the toes of your right foot off the floor.

ADVANCED

After completing 1 set of this move, immediately assume the T Pose (see page 201). Then switch legs.

ORIGINAL MOVE

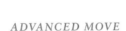

ADVANCED MOVE

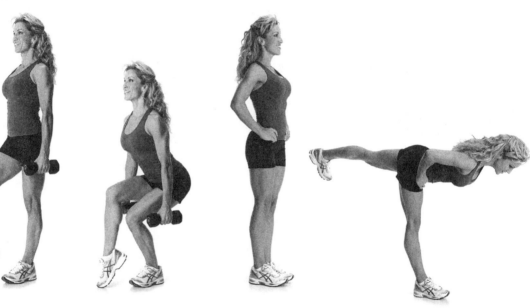

USE YOUR HEAD

To perform moves on a narrow balance beam, a gymnast must plant her foot on the beam and contract every single muscle in her core. Picture yourself performing this move on a balance beam. Take your time, and execute the move with grace.

SUGGESTED STRETCH

Moving Flexibility:
Split Leg
(page 34)

Minna Says

Strong muscles begin with strong desire—the desire to challenge one's limits and exceed one's goals.

✤

REVERSE PLANK WITH LEG LIFT

This move—a lift with a unique twist—will really blast your booty.
It also develops core strength, firms the glutes, and tones the hamstrings and back.

SETS AND REPS

BEGINNER: 1 to 2 sets,
no leg lift (see below)
INTERMEDIATE: 2 to 3 sets,
16 to 24 alternating repetitions
ADVANCED: 3 sets,
16 to 24 alternating repetitions

STARTING POSITION

Sit tall on your sit bones with your arms
at your sides and your palms on the floor
by the sides of your butt. Extend your legs
straight out in front of you. Contract your
abdominal muscles and draw your shoulders back and down. Using your core
muscles and glutes, press into your hands
and the backs of your heels and lift your
pelvis until your body becomes one long,
straight line from your head to your heels.

THE MOVE

From the starting position, lift your left
leg, pressing into your right heel as you do
so. Lift your leg as high as you can while
still maintaining good form. Return to the
starting position and perform the move
with your right leg. Continue alternating
reps until you complete 1 set.

FOCUS ON FORM

✤ Elongate your body from your head to
   your heels.
✤ Keep your abs tight to maintain the
   long line position.
✤ Lift your leg only as high as you can
   without twisting, turning, or lowering
   your torso.

AT HOME/AT THE GYM

AT HOME: Perform the move as described.
If you own a stability ball, try the move
below.
AT THE GYM: Try a straight-leg Bridge on
the stability ball. Lie on your back with
your feet on the ball and your knees soft.
Use your glutes to lift your pelvis off the
floor. Return to the starting position.
Repeat until you complete 1 set.

BEGINNER

Build your strength: Try holding the move
for 10 to 30 seconds at a time. Or try it on
the bottom step of a staircase—place your
hands on the step, your feet on the floor.
The extra height makes holding the position a bit easier.

INTERMEDIATE

Instead of lifting your leg straight up and
down, bend your left knee until it's over
your left hip, then straighten the leg, keeping it over your hip. Lower your left leg;
switch legs. Continue alternating reps until you complete 1 set.

ADVANCED

Perform the move as directed, but before
you lower your left leg, lower your pelvis
until it almost (but not quite) touches the
floor. Lift your pelvis again, then lower
your left leg. Switch legs. Continue,
alternating reps, until you complete 1 set.

ORIGINAL MOVE

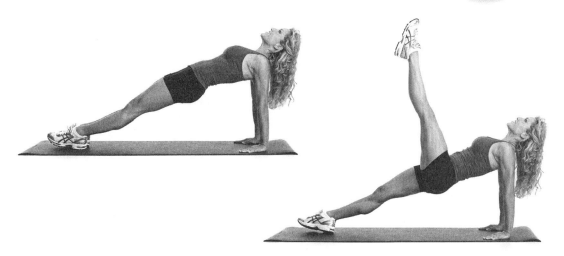

ADVANCED MOVE

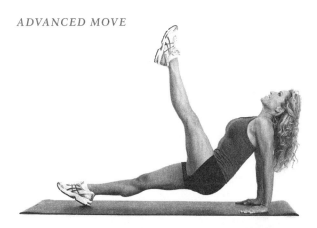

USE YOUR HEAD
The Radio City Music Hall Rockettes keep their cores immobile as they perform their world-famous "kick line." As you perform this move, imagine each lift as a perfectly executed Rockette kick.

BREATHWORK
Exhale as you lift your leg. Inhale as you lower it. If it's hard to balance and breathe rhythmically, simply breathe deep, continual breaths as you balance.

SUGGESTED STRETCH
Static:
Seated Forward Bend
(page 23)

WALKING LUNGE

This total body move will give you glutes of steel.
It sculpts the glutes, tones the quads, and improves balance.

SETS AND REPS

BEGINNER: 1 to 2 sets,
16 to 24 alternating lunges,
no weight or 8-pound dumbbells
INTERMEDIATE: 2 to 3 sets,
16 to 24 alternating lunges,
8- to 12-pound dumbbells
ADVANCED: 3 sets, 18 to 24 alternating
lunges, 12- to 25-pound dumbbells

STARTING POSITION

Hold the dumbbells at your sides with
your palms facing inward. (If you're not
using dumbbells, place your hands on
your hips.) Stand with your feet together.
Contract your abdominal muscles, square
your shoulders and hips, and draw your
shoulders back and down.

THE MOVE

Take a giant step forward with your left
foot. Bend your left knee and lower yourself until your left thigh is parallel with the
floor. Pressing into your left heel, return to
the starting position. Repeat the move,
this time stepping forward with your right
foot. Continue, alternating repetitions,
until you complete 1 set.

Minna Says
If you do only what
you know, you won't do
much. If you try to do
what you don't know,
you'll do more than
you ever dreamed
possible.

FOCUS ON FORM

✤ Perform this move slowly; rushing will
  affect your form.
✤ Contract your abdominal muscles to
  help you maintain your balance.
✤ Keep your chest lifted by drawing your
  shoulders back and down, especially as
  you step forward. Keep your torso
  upright and your spine elongated; avoid
  leaning back or rounding too far
  forward.

AT HOME/AT THE GYM

AT HOME: Try a front/back lunge. Perform the move, stepping forward with
your right leg. Instead of alternating legs,
however, step backward with your right
leg into a reverse lunge (see page 184).
AT THE GYM: Try the front/back lunge on
a Bosu ball. Place your right foot at the
center of the ball and perform the move.
This variation is for intermediate and
advanced readers only.

BEGINNER

Use no weight until you master the form
and can maintain your balance with each
step.

INTERMEDIATE

Instead of stopping between every repetition, go right into the next lunge without
bringing your feet back together. For example, lunge forward with your left foot.
As you stand to return to starting position,
lift your right foot and immediately move
into the right-leg lunge. Continue alternating until you complete 1 set.

ADVANCED

Add a Hip Extension (see page 170): Perform the move as directed. As you return to the starting position, lift your left (back) leg behind you, then sweep your left leg forward directly into a lunge. As you stand back up, lift your right leg behind you. Continue, alternating repetitions, until you complete 1 set.

ORIGINAL MOVE

ADVANCED MOVE

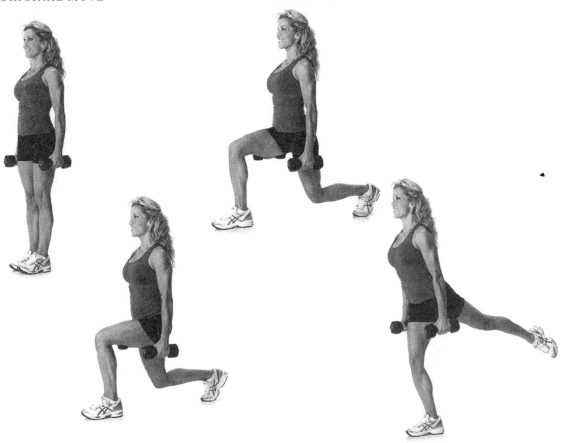

USE YOUR HEAD

Think of this move as the "catwalk" of fitness. Perform the move with a model's even, steady pace and your eyes trained straight ahead.

BREATHWORK

Inhale as you step forward into the lunge. Exhale as you return to the starting position.

SUGGESTED STRETCH

Static:
Kneeling Lunge (page 25)
Moving Flexibility:
Split Leg (page 34)

PART 4

PUTTING IT ALL
Together

In the chapters that follow, I've included three programs—one for each fitness level. Each will challenge and tone your body for lasting results.

THE NOVICE PROGRAM *is for you if you are completely new to exercise or if you have not exercised in at least 1 year.*

THE SKILLED PROGRAM *is for you if you have completed the Novice Program and can execute those moves with good form, if you have lifted weights on your own or with a trainer for at least 6 months, or if you're fit but not ready for the Master Program.*

THE MASTER PROGRAM *is for you if you have a clear understanding of form and perform movements with correct technique; if you are experienced in executing basic fitness moves (squats, lunges, pushups, shoulder presses) and have the strength and flexibility to take on challenging, nontraditional weight-bearing exercise; or if you have been working out for some time and feel you need an extra push to get results.*

10

NOVICE LEVEL:
4-WEEK TOTAL BODY PROGRAM

Welcome, Novices! Making the decision to become fitter and healthier is worthy of big applause. Now, for a few words of wisdom.

It's tempting to go hard and give it your all right off the bat. Whether you're just unaware of how much is too much or you're filled with enthusiasm and think more is better, I urge you to proceed at a slow, comfortable pace. Train cautiously during your 1st week, paying close attention to how you feel. Taking your time during these first workouts allows your body to get used to the idea of moving and to experience being challenged as pleasurable, rather than punishing.

Expect your muscles to feel a tiny bit sore—the kind of soreness that eases with gentle massage, rather than the kind that makes you wince when you're walking down the stairs or getting into your car. If you become very sore right off the bat, you're apt to take too much time off to recover or, worse, be turned off by working out. So, take it easy.

Your focus should be on form, form, and form. If you do not use proper form, you will not get good results. Worse, you may injure your muscles. But the good news is that, as a beginner, you can learn correct form right from the start and build a strong foundation. If you're working out at home, consider investing in a full-length mirror so you can watch yourself as you train and adjust your form as you go along.

If some of the moves feel difficult, take heart—they're supposed to be. The body always tries to find the easy way out by using other muscles to assist the ones being targeted. Good technique challenges the body, and when you use it your muscles will adapt to their increased workload in just a few weeks.

Have patience with your body. Although your mind might understand how to perform the move, your body may need some practice to really grasp it. And above all, stay positive in your attitude. Realize that every effort—small or big—counts toward achieving your goals. So encourage yourself, congratulate yourself, cheer yourself on!

In addition, follow these tips as you work your way through the program.

❖ After 4 weeks, you may repeat the program, or move on to the Skilled Program if you feel you're ready.

❖ If you choose to move on to the Skilled Program and any of the moves prove too challenging, perform the Beginner modification instead.

❖ Perform the stretching exercises that accompany most moves. Taking 30 seconds to stretch between sets increases bloodflow to the working muscles, supplying them with the oxygen and nutrients needed for the next set. These stretches will also help alleviate muscle soreness.

❖ Fill your water bottle before your workout and sip from it frequently.

❖ In addition to this program, perform at least three 30-minute cardio workouts per week, either on the same days as your training or on "off" days. If you don't have 30 minutes to spare, break your cardio session into two or three 10- to 15-minute segments.

❖ Recover as hard as you train. Eating moderate portions of healthy foods (see page 263 for more on proper nutrition), hydrating properly, sleeping sufficiently, and having a positive attitude all contribute to recovering quickly. Also, a warm bath can soothe muscle soreness like nothing else can!

THE PROGRAM

During Weeks 1 and 3, you will train four times per week; during Weeks 2 and 4, you will train three times per week, resting 1 day between workouts. If this schedule proves too intense, you may train three times per week every week, resting at least 1 day between workouts. However, you will not get the same results.

Novices, you will perform the Total Body Workout (TBW), a shuffling of the upper body, lower body, and core moves. You can do the TBW in a circuit—completing 1 set of the first move, then 1 set of the second move, and so on, and repeating the circuit if you feel up to it—or you can perform 2 sets of each move and then progress to the next move. For example, you would perform 2 sets of move 1, then 2 sets of move 2, and so on.

WEEK 1	WEEK 2	WEEK 3	WEEK 4
MONDAY	**MONDAY**	**MONDAY**	**MONDAY**
Total Body Workout	No workout	Total Body Workout	No workout
TUESDAY	**TUESDAY**	**TUESDAY**	**TUESDAY**
No workout	Total Body Workout	No workout	Total Body Workout
WEDNESDAY	**WEDNESDAY**	**WEDNESDAY**	**WEDNESDAY**
Total Body Workout	No workout	Total Body Workout	No workout
THURSDAY	**THURSDAY**	**THURSDAY**	**THURSDAY**
No workout	Total Body Workout	No workout	Total Body Workout
FRIDAY	**FRIDAY**	**FRIDAY**	**FRIDAY**
Total Body Workout	No workout	Total Body Workout	No workout
SATURDAY	**SATURDAY**	**SATURDAY**	**SATURDAY**
No workout	Total Body Workout	No workout	Total Body Workout
SUNDAY	**SUNDAY**	**SUNDAY**	**SUNDAY**
Total Body Workout	No workout	Total Body Workout	No workout

THE MOVES

I've grouped the exercises into three difficulty levels—easy, moderate, and challenging—for you to choose from, with three alternate routines for each level. You can also select which of two sequences to perform them in over the course of the program.

OPTION 1: Start your week with Workout A routines (easy) and end it with Workout C routines (challenging). For example, perform Workout A routines on Mondays, Workout B routines on Wednesdays, and Workout C routines on Fridays.

OPTION 2: Perform Workout A routines during Week 1, alternate between a Workout A and a Workout B routine during Weeks 2 and 3, and graduate to the Workout C routines for Week 4.

♣ TOTAL BODY WORKOUT A (EASY)

WORKOUT A : OPTION 1

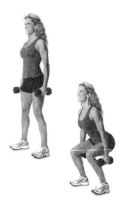

1. SQUAT

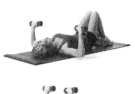
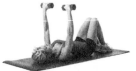

2. LEG LIFT

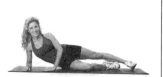
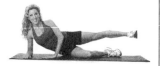

3. CHEST PRESS

WORKOUT A : OPTION 2

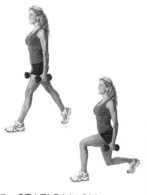

1. STATIONARY LUNGE

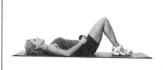
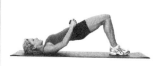

2. BRIDGE

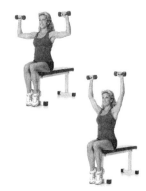

3. SHOULDER PRESS

WORKOUT A : OPTION 3

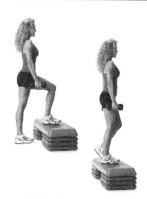

1. STEP-UP

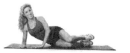
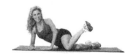
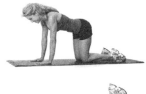
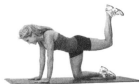

2. HIP EXTENSION

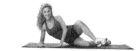

3. KNEE/HEEL TAP

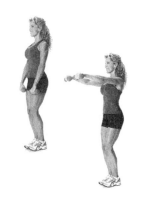

4. FRONT RAISE

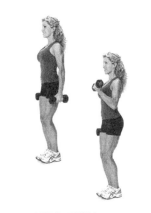

5. BICEPS CURL

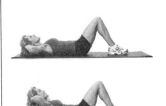

6. 1-2-3 CRUNCH!

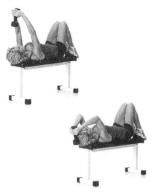

4. LYING TRICEPS
EXTENSION

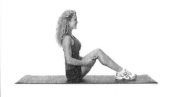

5. BOAT POSE

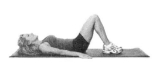

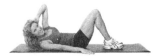

6. BASIC
OBLIQUE TWIST

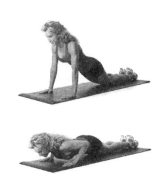

4. MODIFIED
PUSHUP

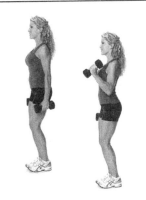

5. HAMMER CURL

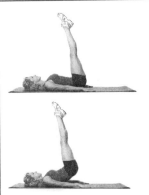

6. DOUBLE
LEG LIFT

✤ TOTAL BODY WORKOUT B (MODERATE)

WORKOUT B : OPTION 1

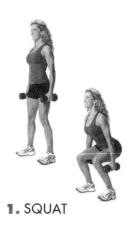

1. SQUAT

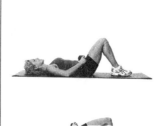

2. BRIDGE

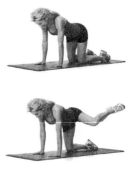

3. LEG ABDUCTION

WORKOUT B : OPTION 2

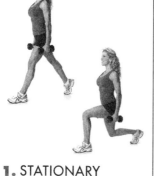

1. STATIONARY LUNGE

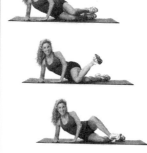

2. KNEE/HEEL TAP

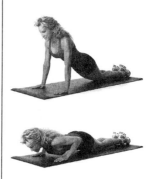

3. MODIFIED PUSHUP

WORKOUT B : OPTION 3

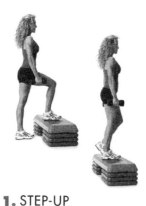

1. STEP-UP

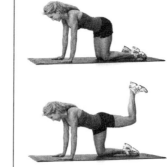

2. HIP EXTENSION

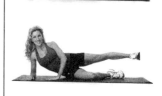

3. LEG LIFT

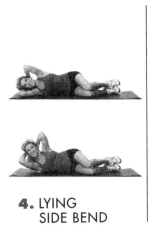

4. LYING
SIDE BEND

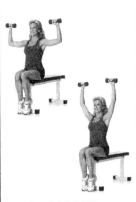

5. SHOULDER
PRESS

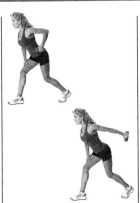

6. TRICEPS
KICKBACK

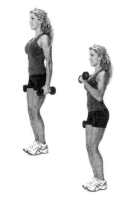

7. BICEPS CURL

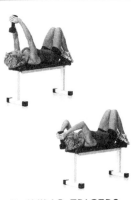

4. LYING TRICEPS
EXTENSION

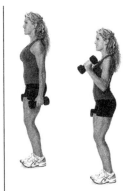

5. HAMMER CURL

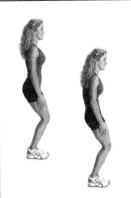

6. FUNKY ABS

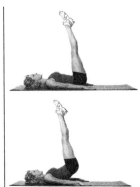

7. DOUBLE
LEG LIFT

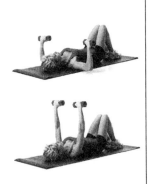

4. CHEST PRESS

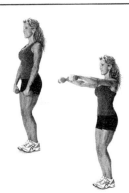

5. FRONT RAISE

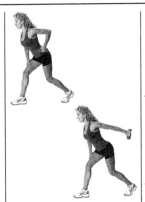

6. TRICEPS
KICKBACK

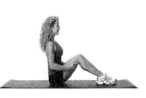
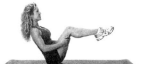

7. BOAT POSE

♣ TOTAL BODY WORKOUT C (CHALLENGING)

WORKOUT C : OPTION 1

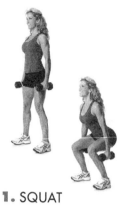 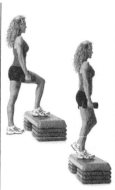 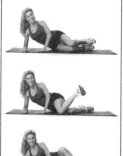 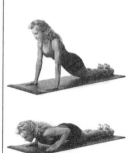

1. SQUAT **2.** STEP-UP **3.** KNEE/ HEEL TAP **4.** MODIFIED PUSHUP

WORKOUT C : OPTION 2

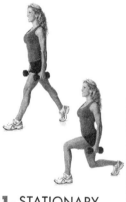 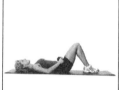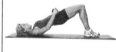 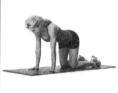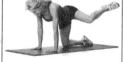 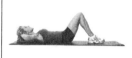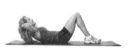

1. STATIONARY LUNGE **2.** BRIDGE **3.** LEG ABDUCTION **4.** BASIC CRUNCH

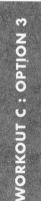

WORKOUT C : OPTION 3

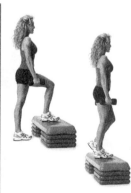 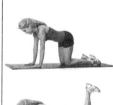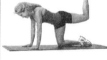 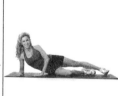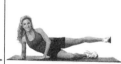 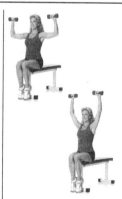

1. STEP-UP **2.** HIP EXTENSION **3.** LEG LIFT **4.** SHOULDER PRESS

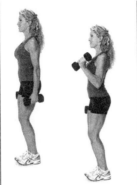
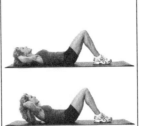
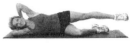
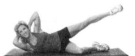
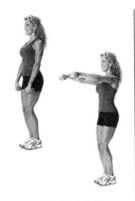

5. FRONT RAISE

6. HAMMER CURL

7. 1-2-3 CRUNCH!

8. LYING SIDE BEND

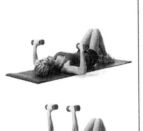
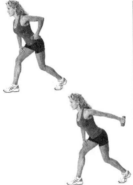
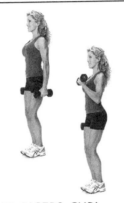
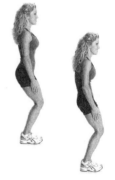

5. CHEST PRESS

6. TRICEPS KICKBACK

7. BICEPS CURL

8. FUNKY ABS

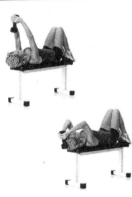
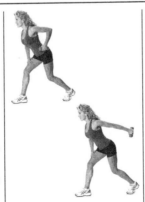
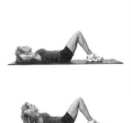
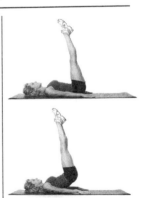

5. LYING TRICEPS EXTENSION

6. TRICEPS KICKBACK

7. BASIC CRUNCH

8. DOUBLE LEG LIFT

INSTANT FITNESS MOTIVATION

Workout boredom, conditioning plateaus, and injuries can all sidetrack your fitness training. But with the right inspiration, you can work through those barriers. When obstacles threaten to keep you from working out, try some of these quick and easy tips to stay on track.

MAKE A DATE. Set up a standing date for exercise with a friend whose fitness level matches yours. The lulls in motivation that you'll both experience will cancel each other out. Research shows that having a dedicated workout partner makes you more likely to stick with an exercise program.

SET A DATE. Accept that invitation to a wedding or high school reunion. Or throw a party 3 months from now—but send out the invitations this week. Anticipating an event at which you'd like to look your best may help you ward off a cookie binge or get moving when you don't feel like it.

PILE ON THE REWARDS. Women tend to save rewards for when they accomplish distant, huge goals, like losing 20 pounds or three dress sizes. Rather than making

3 KEYS TO BEGINNER SUCCESS

❖ Try to train at the time of day when your energy level is at its peak and you won't be rushed or distracted. Try to limit rest time between sets to 60 to 90 seconds. During this time, stretch, sip your water, and tell yourself, "Keep up the good work!"

❖ Wear comfortable workout clothing that feels good and moves freely with your body (nothing constricting!). Clothing made with breathable fabrics that wick away sweat is great—it will keep you feeling comfortable well into your workout. Also, wear a good pair of sneakers suited to your feet's anatomy (shoes with a supportive arch if you have flat feet, for example). If you're shopping for new sneakers, ask a salesperson at a reputable sporting goods store for advice on the right pair for you.

❖ Play your favorite music as you train. Music instantly boosts motivation. How can you not want to move when you're listening to your favorite tunes? If music doesn't work, try listening to a book on tape. Anything pleasurable that you can link to exercise will help motivate you.

goals destination-dependent, make them behavior-dependent. Set a goal, and when you achieve it, give yourself a nonfood reward, like the new issue of a glossy magazine or new nail polish. Pick little indulgences you wouldn't ordinarily give yourself.

DON'T LET STRESS GO TO YOUR HEAD (OR THIGHS)

Next time you have a bad day at work or a fight with your spouse, or are just being pulled in too many directions, try one of these stress busters instead of raiding the fridge.

1. **BREATHE.** When we're tense, we tend to hold our breath or breathe shallowly, which only increases our stress. The next time you feel like you're about to lose it, inhale deeply through your nose. At the top of the breath, expand your lungs even more. Then, exhale slowly through your nose, continuing even after you think you've blown out all your breath. After two or three deep breaths, you should feel quite a bit calmer.

2. **TAKE A ZEN-MINUTE BREAK.** Retreat to a quiet room or close your office door, close your eyes, and silently chant a calming word that appeals to you, such as "peace." Or consider silently reciting the Serenity Prayer: "Grant me the serenity to accept the things I cannot change, courage to change the things I can, and wisdom to know the difference."

3. **SMILE.** A smile is an instant spiritual pick-me-up. When you're about to crack, crack a grin instead. It's virtually impossible to let stress get the best of you when you're smiling.

4. **TALK IT OUT.** Sometimes what appears to be a big ordeal to us is miraculously solved after talking it out with a trusted loved one or friend. When you feel overwhelmed, overtaxed, over-anything—a little opening up can do wonders.

5. **GET OUT IN NATURE.** The gentle swaying of windblown trees or the meandering of a stream can slow body rhythms that have built to a stress-induced peak.

11

SKILLED LEVEL:
4-WEEK UPPER AND LOWER BODY PROGRAM

Welcome to the Skilled Program! For the next 4 weeks, you'll continue shaping and toning your body by combining the moves you learned in the Novice Program—which you'll still do—with more-complicated exercises, thus challenging your mind as well as your muscles.

The Skilled Program includes fun new moves such as the Roll Back and Reach (see page 138) and the Walking Plank (see page 130) that take your muscles to the next level of training. It also emphasizes training your core musculature—not just your abs, but your chest, sides, groin, and upper back—which will balance your body with increased strength and flexibility from inside (your deepest layers of muscle) out (the muscles you see). The result of that balance: pleasing symmetry and proportions.

Follow these tips as you work your way through the program.

❖ After you have completed this program, you may repeat it, or move on to the Master Program if you feel you're ready.

❖ If any move is too challenging, perform the Beginner modification instead.

❖ Perform the stretching exercises that accompany most moves. Taking 30 seconds to stretch between sets increases bloodflow to the working muscles, supplying them with the oxygen and nutrients needed for the next set. These stretches will help alleviate muscle soreness, too.

✤ In addition to this program, perform at least three 30-minute cardio workouts per week, either on the same days as your training or on "off" days. As in the Novice Program, if you don't have 30 minutes, try to squeeze in two or three sessions of 10 or 15 minutes each.

✤ Before you start working out, fill your water bottle, and sip from it frequently.

Let's get started!

THE PROGRAM

For the first 2 weeks, you'll work out 4 days a week, performing two upper body workouts and two lower body workouts in alternating fashion. Follow my suggestions below, or alternate as you choose.

WEEKS 1 & 2

ROTATION OPTION 1	ROTATION OPTION 2	ROTATION OPTION 3	ROTATION OPTION 4
MONDAY	**MONDAY**	**MONDAY**	**MONDAY**
Upper Body Workout	Lower Body Workout	Lower Body Workout	Upper Body Workout
TUESDAY	**TUESDAY**	**TUESDAY**	**TUESDAY**
Lower Body Workout	No workout	Upper Body Workout	No workout
WEDNESDAY	**WEDNESDAY**	**WEDNESDAY**	**WEDNESDAY**
No workout	Upper Body Workout	No workout	Lower Body Workout
THURSDAY	**THURSDAY**	**THURSDAY**	**THURSDAY**
Upper Body Workout	No workout	Lower Body Workout	No workout
FRIDAY	**FRIDAY**	**FRIDAY**	**FRIDAY**
Lower Body Workout	Lower Body Workout	Upper Body Workout	Upper Body Workout
SATURDAY	**SATURDAY**	**SATURDAY**	**SATURDAY**
No workout	Upper Body Workout	No workout	No workout
SUNDAY	**SUNDAY**	**SUNDAY**	**SUNDAY**
No workout	No workout	No workout	Lower Body Workout

WEEK 3	WEEK 4
MONDAY	**MONDAY**
Upper Body Workout	Lower Body Workout
TUESDAY	**TUESDAY**
Lower Body Workout	Upper Body Workout
WEDNESDAY	**WEDNESDAY**
No workout	No workout
THURSDAY	**THURSDAY**
Upper Body Workout	Lower Body Workout
FRIDAY	**FRIDAY**
Lower Body Workout	Upper Body Workout
SATURDAY	**SATURDAY**
No workout	No workout
SUNDAY	**SUNDAY**
Upper Body Workout	Lower Body Workout

THE MOVES

For this program, I've selected moves from both the Novice and Skilled levels. The moves marked with an asterisk (*) are described in the "Novice" section of the book, but for this program, you should perform the Intermediate or Advanced modification.

You can work your way methodically through the list two or three times, so that you perform 1 set of each move and then advance to the next move, or perform 2 or 3 sets of each move before progressing to the next move.

As the week progresses, increase your workout's level of intensity—that is, start with a relatively easy level of exertion on Monday and really challenge yourself by the end of the week. If you go in blazing on Monday and get sore in the next day or two, you are more apt to skip a workout. Another reason to schedule your most challenging workouts for the week's end is that chances are you'll have more time to rest and sleep over the weekend. Sleep is a critical factor in muscle recovery.

If you work out on 2 consecutive days, select a different workout each day to prevent boredom and target your muscles most effectively.

♣ UPPER BODY WORKOUT A (EASY)

WORKOUT A : OPTION 1

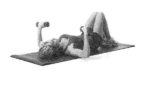
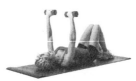

1. CHEST PRESS

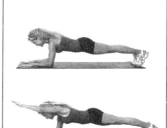

2. MODIFIED PLANK

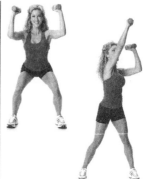

3. ROTATIONAL SHOULDER PRESS

WORKOUT A : OPTION 2

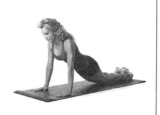
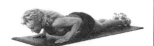

1. MODIFIED PUSHUP

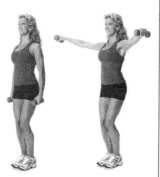

2. LATERAL RAISE

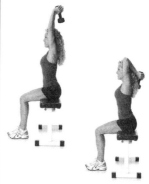

3. OVERHEAD TRICEPS EXTENSION

WORKOUT A : OPTION 3

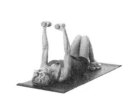
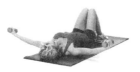

1. CHEST FLY

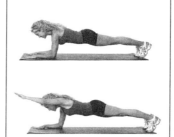

2. MODIFIED PLANK

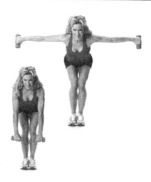

3. REAR DELTOID FLY

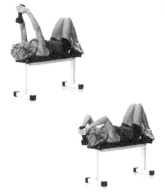

4. LYING TRICEPS EXTENSION

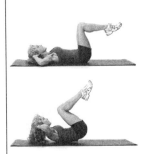

5. BICEPS CURL

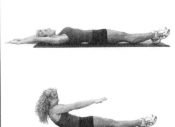

6. TOTAL BODY CRUNCH

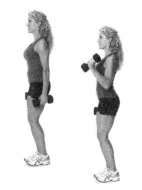

4. HAMMER CURL

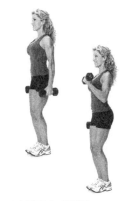

5. ROLL-UP

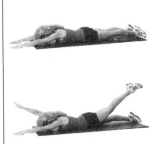

6. SUPERMAN

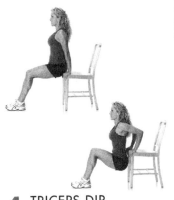

4. TRICEPS DIP

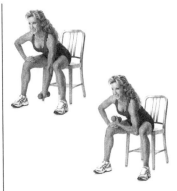

5. CONCENTRATION CURL

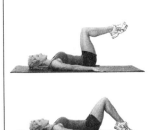

6. DIPPING TOES IN WATER

♣ UPPER BODY WORKOUT B (MODERATE)

WORKOUT B : OPTION 1

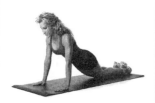
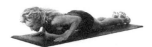
1. MODIFIED PUSHUP

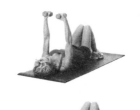
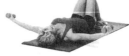
2. CHEST FLY

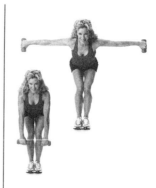
3. REAR DELTOID FLY

WORKOUT B : OPTION 2

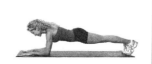
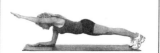
1. MODIFIED PLANK

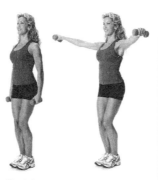
2. LATERAL RAISE

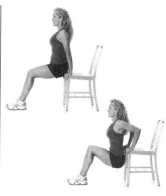
3. TRICEPS DIP

WORKOUT B : OPTION 3

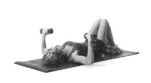
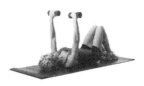
1. CHEST PRESS

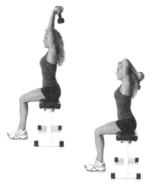
2. OVERHEAD TRICEPS EXTENSION

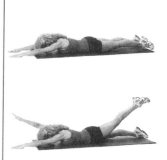
3. SUPERMAN

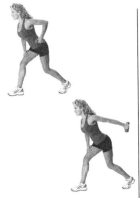

4. TRICEPS
KICKBACK

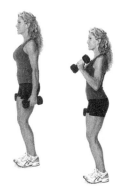

5. HAMMER CURL

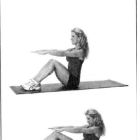

6. ROLL BACK
AND REACH

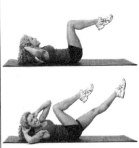

7. BICYCLE

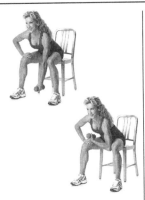

4. CONCENTRA-
TION CURL

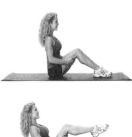

5. BOAT POSE

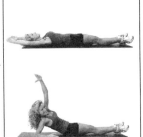

6. BALLERINA
TWIST

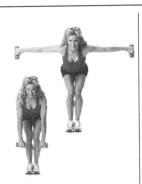

4. REAR
DELTOID FLY

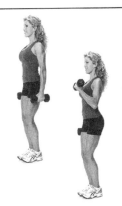

5. BICEPS CURL

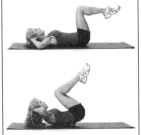

6. TOTAL BODY
CRUNCH

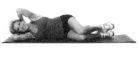
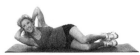

7. LYING
SIDE BEND

♣ UPPER BODY WORKOUT C (CHALLENGING)

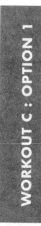

WORKOUT C : OPTION 1

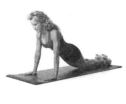

1. MODIFIED PUSHUP

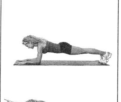

2. MODIFIED PLANK

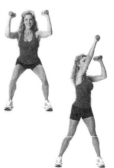

3. ROTATIONAL SHOULDER PRESS

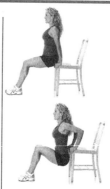

4. TRICEPS DIP

WORKOUT C : OPTION 2

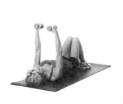

1. CHEST FLY

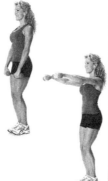

2. *FRONT RAISE

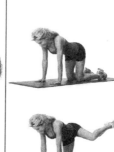

3. LEG ABDUCTION

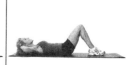
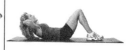

4. BASIC CRUNCH

WORKOUT C : OPTION 3

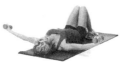
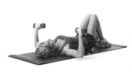

1. *CHEST PRESS

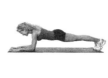
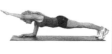

2. MODIFIED PLANK

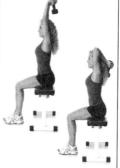

3. OVERHEAD TRICEPS EXTENSION

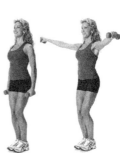

4. LATERAL RAISE

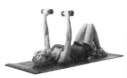

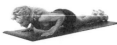

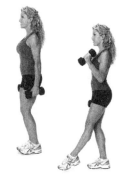

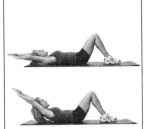

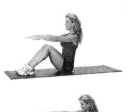

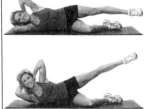

5. *HAMMER CURL

6. *1-2-3 CRUNCH!

7. ROLL BACK AND REACH

8. *LYING SIDE BEND

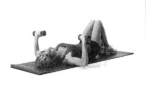

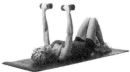

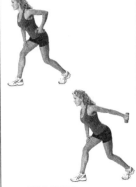

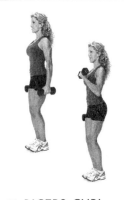

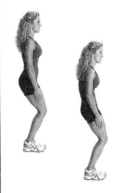

5. CHEST PRESS

6. TRICEPS KICKBACK

7. BICEPS CURL

8. FUNKY ABS

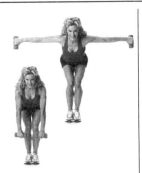

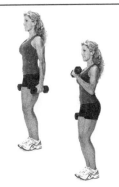

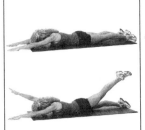

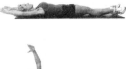

5. REAR DELTOID FLY

6. BICEPS CURL

7. SUPERMAN

8. BALLERINA TWIST

♣ LOWER BODY WORKOUT A (EASY)

WORKOUT A : OPTION 1

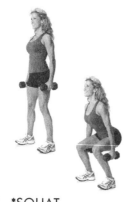

1. *SQUAT

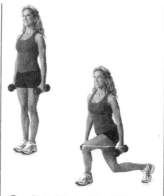

2. CURTSY LUNGE

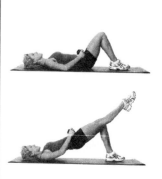

3. *BRIDGE

WORKOUT A : OPTION 2

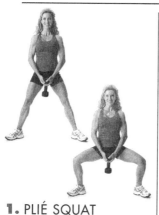

1. PLIÉ SQUAT

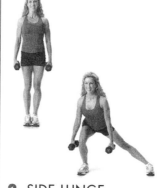

2. SIDE LUNGE

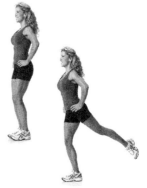

3. STANDING HIP EXTENSION

WORKOUT A : OPTION 3

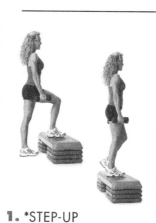

1. *STEP-UP

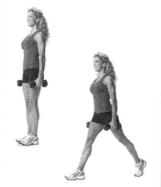

2. ALTERNATING REVERSE LUNGE

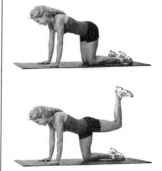

3. *HIP EXTENSION

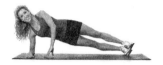
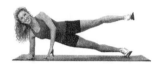

4. *LEG LIFT

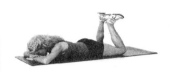
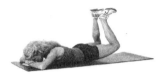

5. FROGGY
DOUBLE-LEG LIFT

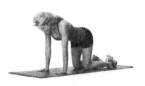
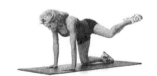

4. *LEG ABDUCTION

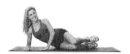
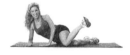
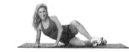

5. *KNEE/HEEL TAP

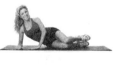
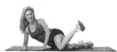
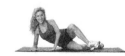

4. *KNEE/HEEL TAP

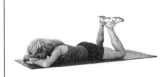
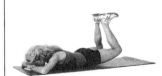

5. FROGGY
DOUBLE-LEG LIFT

♣ LOWER BODY WORKOUT B (MODERATE)

WORKOUT B : OPTION 1

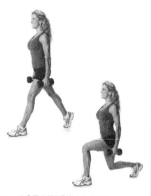

1. *STATIONARY LUNGE

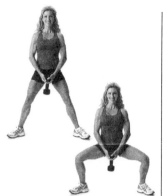

2. PLIÉ SQUAT

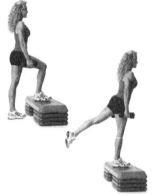

3. *STEP-UP

WORKOUT B : OPTION 2

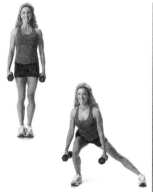

1. SIDE LUNGE

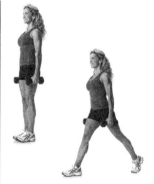

2. ALTERNATING REVERSE LUNGE

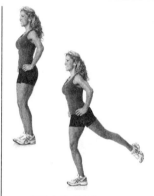

3. STANDING HIP EXTENSION

WORKOUT B : OPTION 3

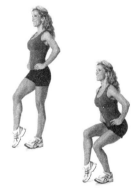

1. *SQUAT

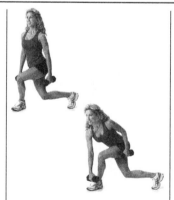

2. *CURTSY LUNGE

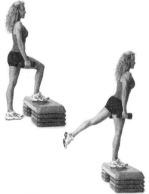

3. *STEP-UP

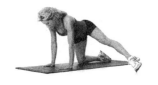
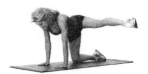

4. *LEG ABDUCTION

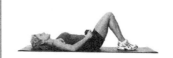
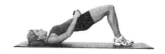

5. BRIDGE

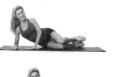
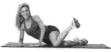
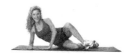

6. *KNEE/HEEL TAP

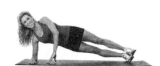

4. *LEG LIFT

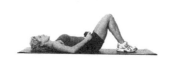
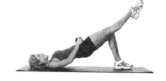

5. *BRIDGE

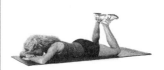

6. FROGGY
DOUBLE-LEG LIFT

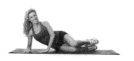
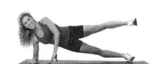
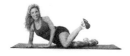
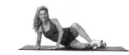

4. *KNEE/HEEL TAP

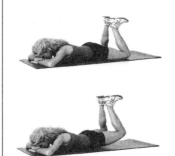

5. FROGGY
DOUBLE-LEG LIFT

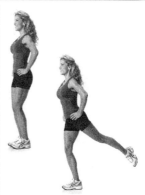

6. STANDING HIP
EXTENSION

♣ LOWER BODY WORKOUT C (CHALLENGING)

WORKOUT C : OPTION 1

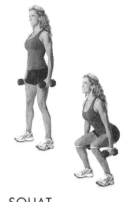

1. SQUAT

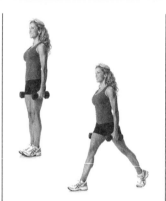

2. ALTERNATING REVERSE LUNGE

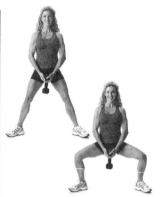

3. PLIÉ SQUAT

WORKOUT C : OPTION 2

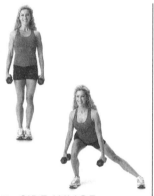

1. SIDE LUNGE

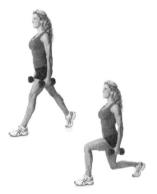

2. *STATIONARY LUNGE

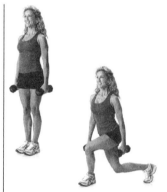

3. CURTSY LUNGE

WORKOUT C : OPTION 3

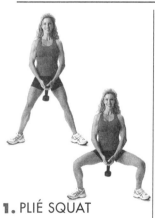

1. PLIÉ SQUAT

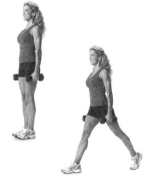

2. ALTERNATING REVERSE LUNGE

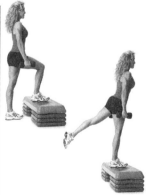

3. *STEP-UP

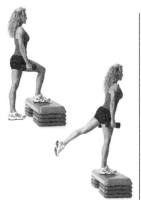

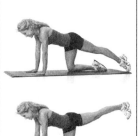

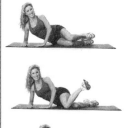

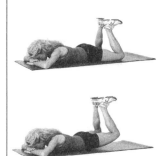

4. *STEP-UP

5. *HIP EXTENSION

6. *KNEE/ HEEL TAP

7. FROGGY DOUBLE-LEG LIFT

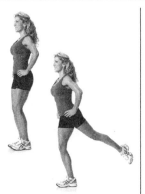

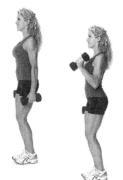

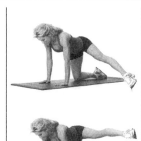

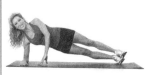

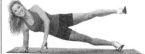

4. STANDING HIP EXTENSION

5. HAMMER CURL

6. *LEG ABDUCTION

7. *LEG LIFT

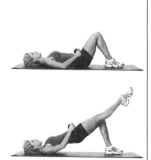

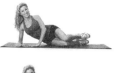

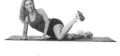

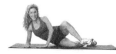

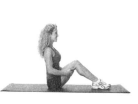

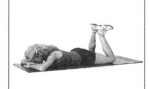

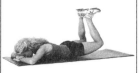

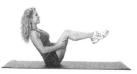

4. *BRIDGE

5. *KNEE/ HEEL TAP

6. FROGGY DOUBLE-LEG LIFT

7. BOAT POSE

14 WAYS TO TAME POSTWORKOUT MUNCHIES

After a workout, your body wants to replenish its fuel, and if you're not careful, you could negate your entire exercise session with one postworkout binge. Luckily, there are smart ways to take the edge off hunger. Use these strategies to squelch an after-workout appetite.

❖ **EASE UP.** Vigorous workouts can rev up your appetite. Researchers at the University of Ottawa found that 13 women consumed enough to replace nearly all the calories they had burned during high-intensity exercise. When they did lower-intensity walking, they had healthy appetites but still netted a 177-calorie deficit for the day.

❖ **SIP MORE.** It's possible to mistake thirst for hunger, so drink before you eat. People who drink about 7 cups of water a day eat nearly 200 fewer calories than those who consume less than a glass a day, report researchers who did a recent study at the University of North Carolina at Chapel Hill.

❖ **EAT WITHIN 30 MINUTES.** Research suggests that working out just before a regularly scheduled meal may help to curb appetite. In studies where meals were served 15 to 30 minutes after exercise, participants were less likely to eat back the calories they'd just burned than were those who had to wait an hour or more to eat.

❖ **REFUEL WISELY.** Can't have a real meal right away? Skip the energy bar and eat a carb-and-protein snack instead, such as 6 ounces of fat-free yogurt with ½ cup of strawberries for just 97 calories.

12

MASTER LEVEL:
4-WEEK FOCUS ON PARTS

Congratulations on having arrived at the Master Program. You have worked hard to get to this point and have made great progress in technique, strength, flexibility, and appearance. I'm proud of you. Now you are ready for the ultimate challenge.

Check your ego at the door of your workout room or gym, however. While you may *think* you know everything there is to know about proper form, you don't. That's okay—I don't, either. In fact, I find that every workout teaches me something new about technique. My advice: Keep your senses attuned and your commitment to technique a priority. Listen to your body more closely than ever—this program will demand your full focus and concentration. Remember, if you don't execute a move flawlessly on the first try, most fitness gurus probably didn't, either. So work at this program with patience and diligence. I know you can do it. You made it here, didn't you?

Follow these tips as you work your way through the program.

❖ After you have completed this program, you may repeat it.

❖ If any move is too challenging, perform the Intermediate modification instead.

✤ Perform the stretching exercises that accompany each move. Taking 30 seconds to stretch between sets increases bloodflow to the working muscles, supplying them with the oxygen and nutrients needed for the next set. These stretches will help alleviate muscle soreness, too.

✤ In addition to this program, perform at least three 30-minute cardio workouts per week, either on the same days as your training or on "off" days. If you don't have 30 minutes to spare, jump on the treadmill or elliptical trainer for 10 or 15 minutes at a time—it's fine to break your cardio workout into two or three segments.

✤ Before you work out, fill your water bottle, and sip from it frequently.

Let's get started!

THE PROGRAM

In Weeks 1 through 4, you will train 6 days per week as follows:

MONDAY: Butt

TUESDAY: Arms

WEDNESDAY: Belly

THURSDAY: No workout

FRIDAY: Butt

SATURDAY: Arms

SUNDAY: Belly

If you find the workouts too intense, you may train only 5 days per week, but you may not get the same results.

THE MOVES

For this program, I've also selected moves from the Beginner and Intermediate levels. I've marked them with an asterisk (*) so you can easily find their descriptions in the relevant sections of the book, but remember to perform their Advanced modification. However, if the Advanced variation is too intense, you can follow the Beginner or Intermediate instructions.

You can work your way methodically through the list two or three times, so that you perform 1 set of each move and then advance to the next move, or perform 2 or 3 sets of each move before progressing to the next move. For example, perform 2 or 3 sets of move 1, 2 or 3 sets of move 2, and so on.

♣ BUTT WORKOUT A (EASY)

WORKOUT A : OPTION 1

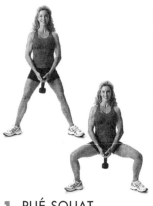

1. PLIÉ SQUAT

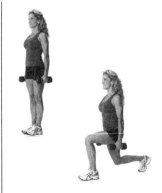

2. WALKING LUNGE

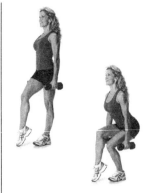

3. ONE-LEGGED SQUAT

WORKOUT A : OPTION 2

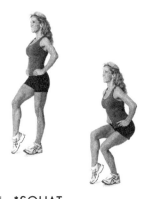

1. *SQUAT

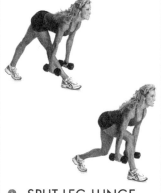

2. SPLIT-LEG LUNGE

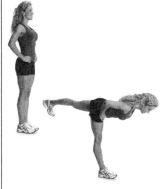

3. T POSE

WORKOUT A : OPTION 3

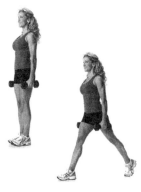

1. ALTERNATING REVERSE LUNGE

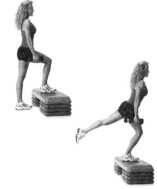

2. *STEP-UP

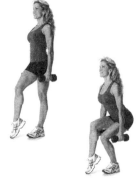

3. ONE-LEGGED SQUAT

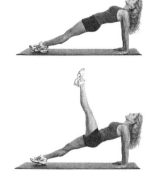
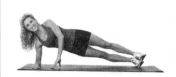
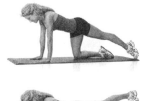

4. REVERSE PLANK
WITH LEG LIFT

5. *LEG LIFT

6. *HIP EXTENSION

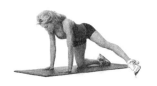
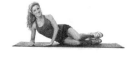
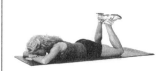

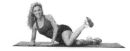
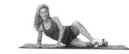
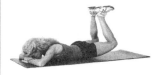

4. *LEG ABDUCTION

5. *KNEE/HEEL TAP

6. FROGGY
DOUBLE-LEG LIFT

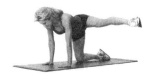
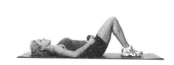
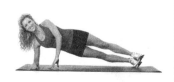
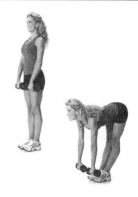

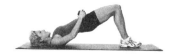
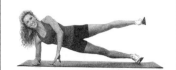

4. BRIDGE

5. *LEG LIFT

6. DEAD LIFT

♣ BUTT WORKOUT B (MODERATE)

WORKOUT B : OPTION 1

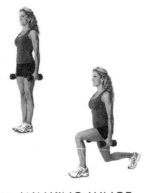

1. WALKING LUNGE

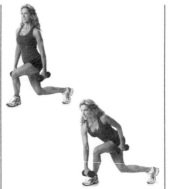

2. *CURTSY LUNGE

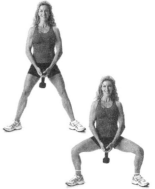

3. PLIÉ SQUAT

WORKOUT B : OPTION 2

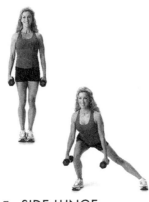

1. SIDE LUNGE

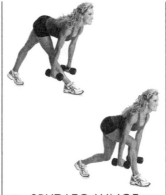

2. SPLIT-LEG LUNGE

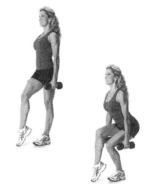

3. ONE-LEGGED SQUAT

WORKOUT B : OPTION 3

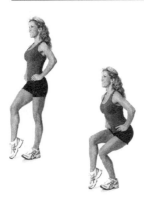

1. *SQUAT

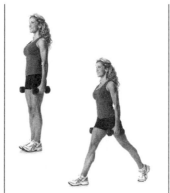

2. ALTERNATING REVERSE LUNGE

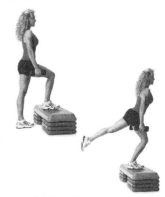

3. *STEP-UP

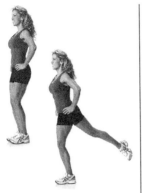

4. STANDING HIP EXTENSION

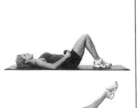

5. *BRIDGE

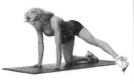

6. *LEG ABDUCTION

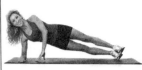
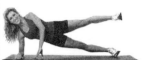

7. *LEG LIFT

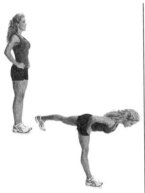

4. T POSE

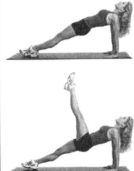

5. REVERSE PLANK WITH LEG LIFT

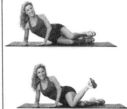
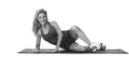

6. KNEE/HEEL TAP

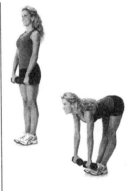

7. DEAD LIFT

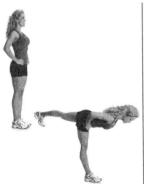

4. T POSE

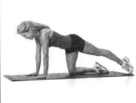

5. *HIP EXTENSION

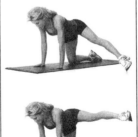

6. *LEG ABDUCTION

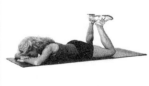
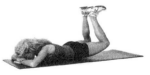

7. FROGGY DOUBLE-LEG LIFT

❖ BUTT WORKOUT C (CHALLENGING)

WORKOUT C : OPTION 1

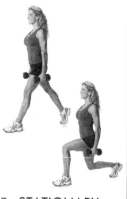 **1. STATIONARY LUNGE**

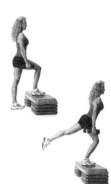 **2. *STEP-UP**

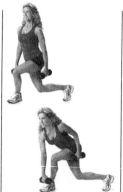 **3. *CURTSY LUNGE**

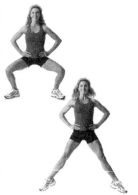 **4. *PLIÉ SQUAT**

WORKOUT C : OPTION 2

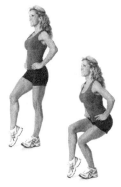 **1. *SQUAT**

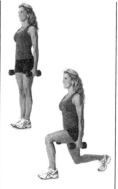 **2. WALKING LUNGE**

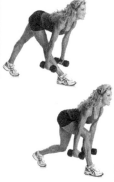 **3. SPLIT-LEG LUNGE**

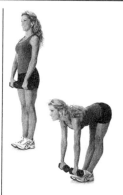 **4. DEAD LIFT**

WORKOUT C : OPTION 3

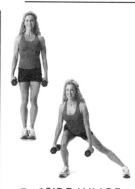 **1. *SIDE LUNGE**

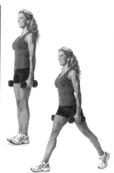 **2. ALTERNAT- ING REVERSE LUNGE**

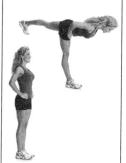 **3. T POSE**

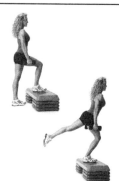 **4. *STEP-UP**

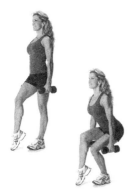

5. ONE-LEGGED SQUAT

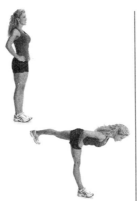

6. T POSE

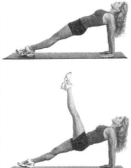

7. REVERSE PLANK WITH LEG LIFT

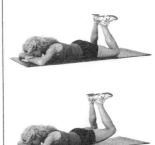

8. *FROGGY DOUBLE-LEG LIFT

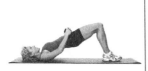
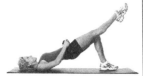

5. *BRIDGE

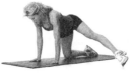
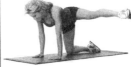

6. *LEG ABDUCTION

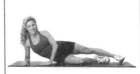
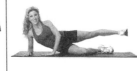

7. LEG LIFT

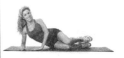
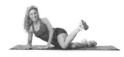
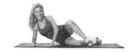

8. KNEE/HEEL TAP

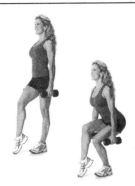

5. ONE-LEGGED SQUAT

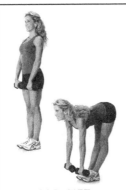

6. DEAD LIFT

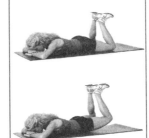

7. FROGGY DOUBLE-LEG LIFT

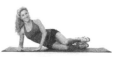
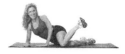
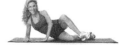

8. KNEE/HEEL TAP

♣ ARMS WORKOUT A (EASY)

WORKOUT A : OPTION 1

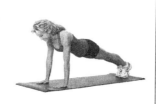
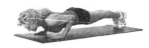

1. YOGI PUSHUP

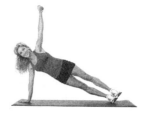
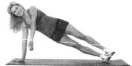

2. *REAR DELTOID FLY

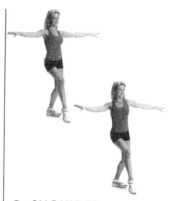

3. SHOULDER SHIMMY

WORKOUT A : OPTION 2

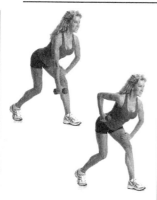

1. BENT-OVER ROW

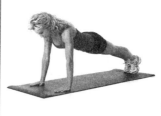
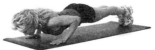

2. *MODIFIED PUSHUP

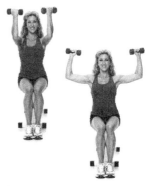

3. ARNOLD PRESS

WORKOUT A : OPTION 3

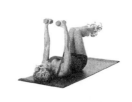
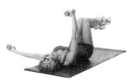

1. *CHEST FLY

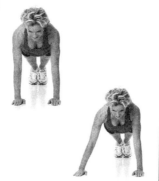

2. PLANK HOLD WALKOUT

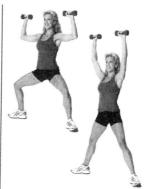

3. *FRONT RAISE

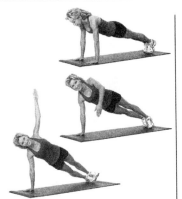

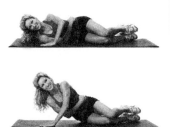

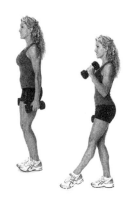

4. FRONT TO
SIDE PLANK

5. ONE-ARM TRICEPS
PUSHUP

6. *HAMMER CURL

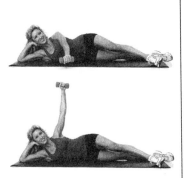

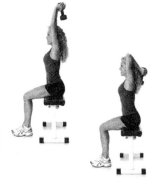

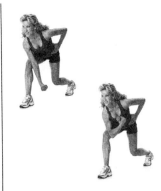

4. *LATERAL RAISE

5. OVERHEAD TRICEPS
EXTENSION

6. CONCENTRATION
CURL

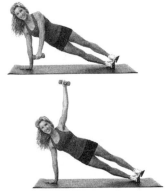

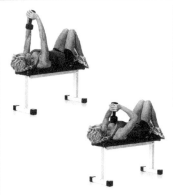

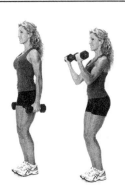

4. SIDE PLANK WITH
ARM RAISE

5. *LYING TRICEPS
EXTENSION

6. *BICEPS CURL

♣ ARMS WORKOUT B (MODERATE)

WORKOUT B : OPTION 1

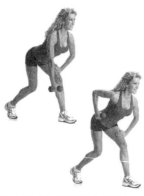

1. BENT-OVER ROW

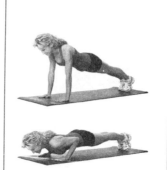

2. YOGI PUSHUP

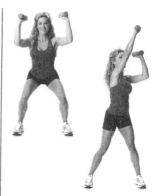

3. *ROTATIONAL SHOULDER PRESS

WORKOUT B : OPTION 2

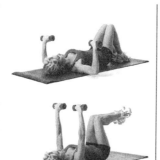

1. *CHEST PRESS

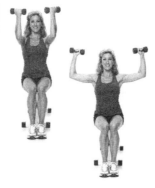

2. ARNOLD PRESS

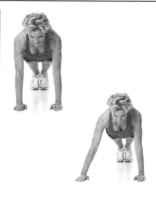

3. PLANK HOLD WALKOUT

WORKOUT B : OPTION 3

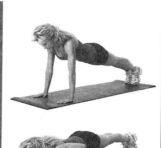

1. *MODIFIED PUSHUP

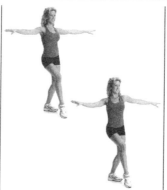

2. SHOULDER SHIMMY

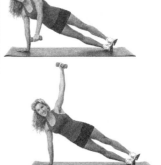

3. SIDE PLANK WITH ARM RAISE

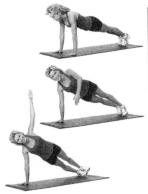 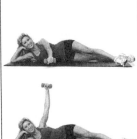 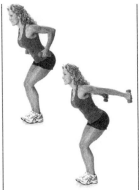 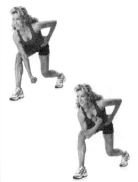

4. FRONT TO
SIDE PLANK

5. *LATERAL
RAISE

6. *TRICEPS
KICKBACK

7. CONCENTRA-
TION CURL

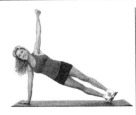 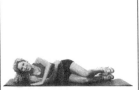 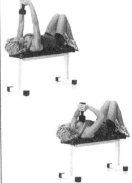 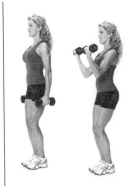
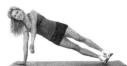 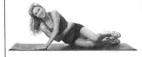

4. *REAR
DELTOID FLY

5. ONE-ARM
TRICEPS PUSHUP

6. *LYING TRICEPS
EXTENSION

7. *BICEPS CURL

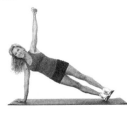 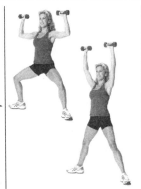 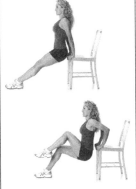 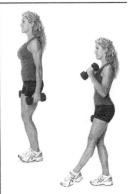
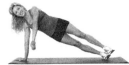

4. *REAR
DELTOID FLY

5. *FRONT RAISE

6. *TRICEPS DIP

7. *HAMMER CURL

♣ ARMS WORKOUT C (CHALLENGING)

WORKOUT C : OPTION 1

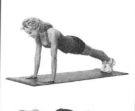
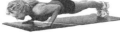

1. YOGI PUSHUP

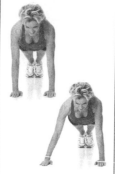

2. PLANK HOLD WALKOUT

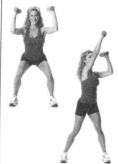

3. *ROTATIONAL SHOULDER PRESS

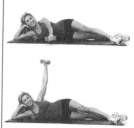

4. *LATERAL RAISE

WORKOUT C : OPTION 2

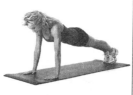

1. *MODIFIED PUSHUP

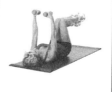
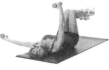

2. *CHEST FLY

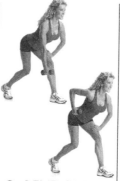

3. BENT-OVER ROW

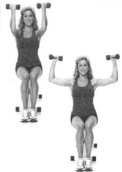

4. ARNOLD PRESS

WORKOUT C : OPTION 3

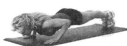
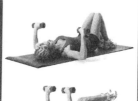
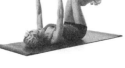

1. *CHEST PRESS

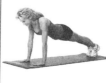
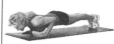

2. YOGI PUSHUP

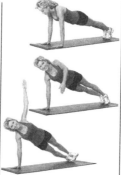

3. FRONT TO SIDE PLANK

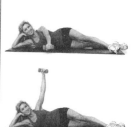

4. *LATERAL RAISE

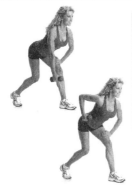

5. BENT-OVER
ROW

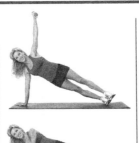

6. *REAR
DELTOID FLY

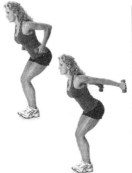

7. *TRICEPS
KICKBACK

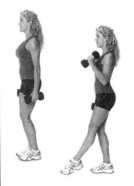

8. *HAMMER CURL

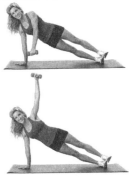

5. SIDE PLANK
WITH ARM
RAISE

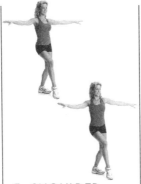

6. SHOULDER
SHIMMY

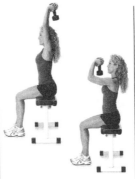

7. *OVERHEAD
TRICEPS
EXTENSION

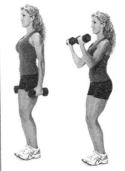

8. *BICEPS CURL

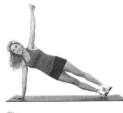
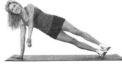

5. *REAR
DELTOID FLY

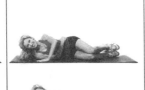

6. ONE-ARM
TRICEPS
PUSHUP

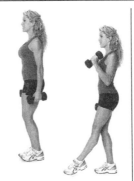

7. *HAMMER CURL

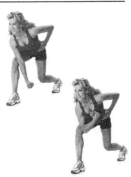

8. *CONCENTRA-
TION CURL

♣ BELLY WORKOUT A (EASY)

WORKOUT A : OPTION 1

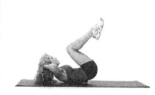
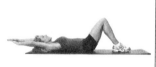

1. *TOTAL BODY CRUNCH

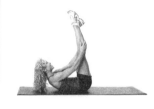
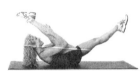

2. SCISSORS

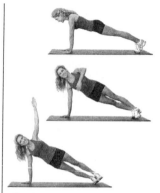
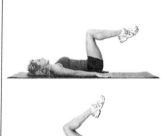

3. SIDE PLANK

WORKOUT A : OPTION 2

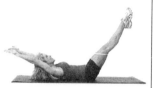
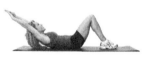

1. *1-2-3 CRUNCH!

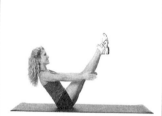
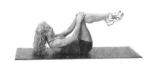

2. *BOAT POSE

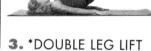

3. *DOUBLE LEG LIFT

WORKOUT A : OPTION 3

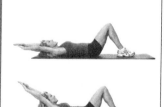

1. *BASIC CRUNCH

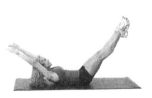

2. ORGAMI CRUNCH

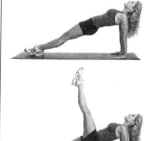

3. REVERSE PLANK

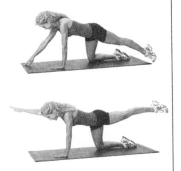

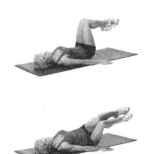

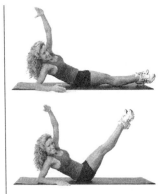

4. ARM AND LEG
EXTENSION

5. KNEE DROP

6. *BALLERINA TWIST

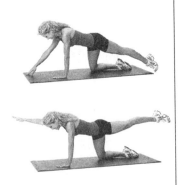

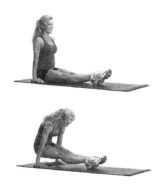

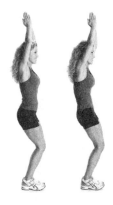

4. *SUPERMAN

5. GYMNAST ABS

6. *FUNKY ABS

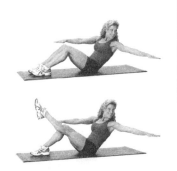

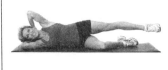

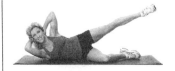

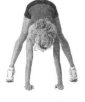

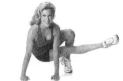

4. *ROLL BACK
AND REACH

5. *LYING SIDE BEND

6. TWIST AND DROP

♣ BELLY WORKOUT B (MODERATE)

WORKOUT B : OPTION 1

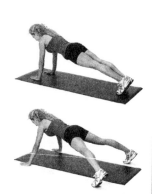

1. *WALKING PLANK

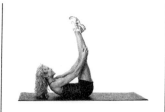
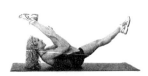

2. SCISSORS

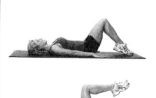
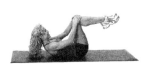

3. DIPPING TOES
IN WATER

WORKOUT B : OPTION 2

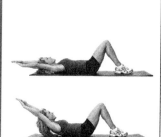

1. *BASIC CRUNCH

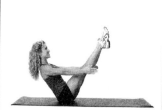

2. BOAT POSE

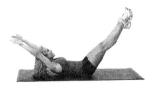

3. ORIGAMI CRUNCH

WORKOUT B : OPTION 3

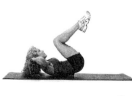
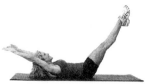

1. *TOTAL
BODY CRUNCH

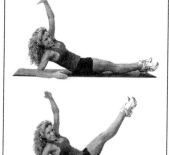

2. *BALLERINA TWIST

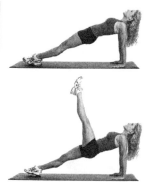

3. REVERSE PLANK

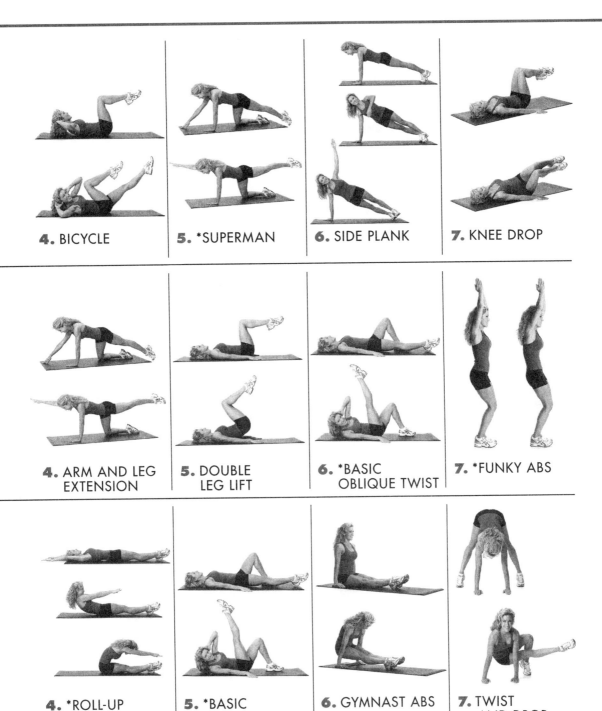

4. BICYCLE

5. *SUPERMAN

6. SIDE PLANK

7. KNEE DROP

4. ARM AND LEG
EXTENSION

5. DOUBLE
LEG LIFT

6. *BASIC
OBLIQUE TWIST

7. *FUNKY ABS

4. *ROLL-UP

5. *BASIC
OBLIQUE TWIST

6. GYMNAST ABS

7. TWIST
AND DROP

♣ BELLY WORKOUT C (CHALLENGING)

WORKOUT C : OPTION 1

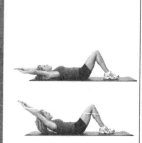

1. *1-2-3 CRUNCH!

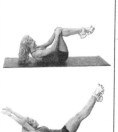

2. ORIGAMI CRUNCH

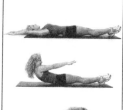

3. *ROLL-UP

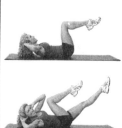

4. *BICYCLE

WORKOUT C : OPTION 2

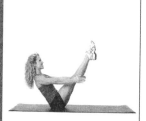

1. *BOAT POSE

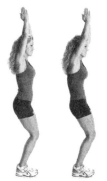

2. *FUNKY ABS

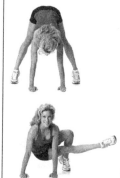

3. TWIST AND DROP

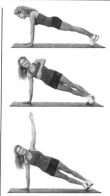

4. SIDE PLANK

WORKOUT C : OPTION 3

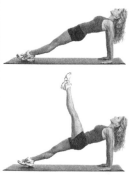

1. REVERSE PLANK

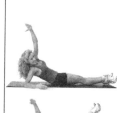
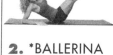

2. *BALLERINA TWIST

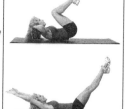

3. *TOTAL BODY CRUNCH

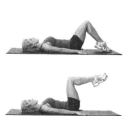

4. DIPPING TOES IN WATER

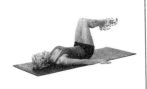
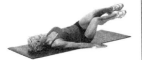

5. KNEE DROP

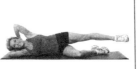
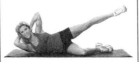

6. *LYING
SIDE BEND

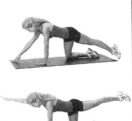

7. *SUPERMAN

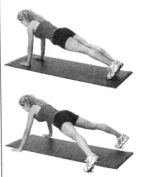

8. *WALKING
PLANK

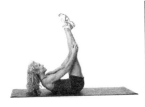
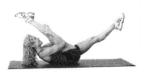

5. SCISSORS

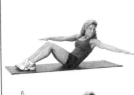
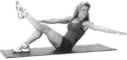

6. *ROLL BACK
AND REACH

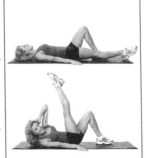

7. *BASIC
OBLIQUE TWIST

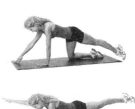

8. ARM AND LEG
EXTENSION

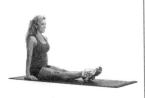
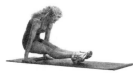

5. GYMNAST ABS

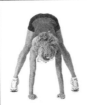
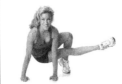

6. TWIST
AND DROP

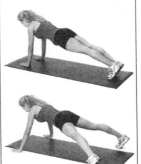

7. *WALKING
PLANK

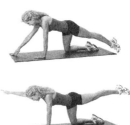

8. *SUPERMAN

❖

STAYING LEAN FOR LIFE:
NUTRITION PRINCIPLES AND PRACTICE

Here's the good news: I'm not putting you on a diet. I won't ask you to count carbo-hydrate or fat grams, drastically curtail your calories to lose body fat, or log every bit of food that passes between your lips (unless you want to).

That's right—you've entered a diet-free zone. Just in time, too. As you probably already know, diets don't work.

How many times have you tried a popular fad diet, lost a few pounds, then gained them all back—and more—when you started eating normally again? Or starved yourself all day only to clean out the fridge or cookie jar at 11 p.m.? These scenarios are just two of the reasons diets don't work. Here are some others.

❖ When you drastically curtail calories, your body thinks it's starving. It hoards fat and burns calorie-burning muscle first. Ironically, at the end of a diet, you have even more body fat than before you started, because diets rob you of muscle.

❖ Dieting robs your brain of fuel, leaving you irritable or in a fog.

❖ Dieting robs your body of fuel, leaving you fatigued.

❖ Numerous studies link chronic dieting with feelings of depression, low self-esteem, and increased stress.

❖ Dieting increases compulsive eating.

You see, diets are temporary. Healthy eating habits are forever. My experience as a personal trainer and fitness competitor has helped me identify certain eating guidelines that will result in peak well-being—a fit mind in a fit body.

Below, you'll find four eating "principles," one for each week of my program. These principles serve as guideposts as you gradually develop new, healthier eating habits. After each week's principle, you'll find a "practice"—a practical way to add new eating habits to your everyday life. As you begin the program, focus on Week 1's principle and practice—no skipping ahead! When you begin Week 2, continue to follow Week 1's guidelines while implementing Week 2's. As you start Week 3, follow the first 2 weeks' guidelines and add in Week 3's. You get the idea. By the end of Week 4, you'll have virtually all the nutrition information you need for getting—and staying—lean and fit for the rest of your life.

Be prepared for a period of adjustment, however. If your taste buds are used to fast-food fried chicken and mashed potatoes and gravy, it will take time for them to accept baked chicken and broccoli without the cheese sauce. But push past this "transition period." After a few weeks, if you allow yourself a less-than-healthy indulgence, chances are that it won't taste quite as good as you'd imagined. This certainly has been my experience. When I was a kid, I loved fast food. In my teens, as I became more conscious of my health and appearance, I cut out the burgers and fries. After a few weeks, I didn't miss them. Recently, I tasted one of my girls' chicken nuggets. *Yuck!* That was my last (and my girls' last!) processed chicken nugget—forever, I hope.

Traditional diets have taught us that to lose weight, we must count calories, keep track of everything we eat, and deprive ourselves by limiting the amount—and kinds—of foods we eat. But losing weight and keeping it off requires a lifestyle change, not a diet "quick fix." I've met so many women who tell me that they've just started this or that new diet. A few have tried virtually every fad diet popularized in the past 15 or 20 years. If this sounds like you, I urge you to start thinking differently. It's my feeling that dieting is a dead-end road—it leads to nothing but frustration. It is far more productive to change your diet gradually, so that you can sustain healthy eating for life.

When you get off the diet roller coaster, you will feel better, become healthier, and lose the weight for good. When the body is well fed with healthy foods, it will shed the extra fat. It doesn't have to store it anymore. And when you give your body the nutrients it needs, you stop craving less-healthy foods.

That said, while I live by these principles, I don't follow them to the extreme. Even when I trained for fitness competitions, I allowed myself an occasional splurge, like a bowl of pasta with Alfredo sauce or a brownie sundae. What is life without the occasional piece of chocolate—or for me, the small bag of sour cream and onion–

WHAT I EAT (AND HOW I CHEAT)

When I became a mom, my eating habits changed drastically. I try my best to eat healthy, but my diet is not perfect. I *need* a handful of sour cream and onion–flavored potato chips around that time of the month. I love sweets, too, so I bake cookies, muffins, and cakes—with fresh fruit, whole grains, and other healthy ingredients—and indulge a few times a week. Pizza is a staple food at my house—my girls love it, and it's fast and easy.

That said, I eat these items in moderation and burn them up with regular exercise. This is very good news, because if I can eat this way, so can you!

Breakfast
BREAKFAST BURRITO: 3 scrambled eggs (2 whites, 1 yolk) wrapped in a whole wheat burrito and topped with a mixture of shredded mozzarella, brown rice, tomatoes, black beans, salsa, and avocado

Snack
6 Triscuits
2 tablespoons peanut butter

Lunch
Turkey sandwich with 1 slice of American cheese on whole grain bread *or* a spinach salad with red, yellow, or orange peppers, lightly steamed asparagus, and topped with chicken or tuna and 2 tablespoons of Ranch or Italian dressing

Snack
1 small homemade muffin *or* a smoothie, made with fresh fruit juice and 1 scoop of protein powder

Dinner
1 serving of chicken or fish, 1 portion of healthy carbohydrate (either whole grain rice, a sweet potato, beans), and salad or steamed veggies

flavored potato chips? Yes, food is fuel, but it's also one of the great pleasures of life. As I write this, I'm eating a sliver of homemade peach pie—a sliver is all you need to satisfy the taste for something decadent—and I don't feel guilty at all. I worked out hard this morning and ate a healthy breakfast and lunch, so I'm thoroughly enjoying every bite. My hope for you is that, like me, you will find a healthy balance between indulgence and nourishment.

WEEK 1
LEAN-FOR-LIFE PRINCIPLE:
LEARN THE DIFFERENCE BETWEEN HUNGER AND APPETITE

If your body could talk, it would tell you exactly what to feed it to attain and maintain a healthy weight. It might ask for cottage cheese and fruit for breakfast. A tuna sandwich on whole grain bread for lunch. A grilled-chicken salad, heavy on the veggies, for dinner. And water—lots and lots of water. If only your body could talk. Right?

It can. You just need to learn how to listen.

I believe that we're on the verge of forgetting our bodies' "language." We live in a society where fast food beckons from every street corner, and exercise has become synonymous with misery. In short, although we live in a culture that worships fitness, we don't treat our bodies with the respect and care that they deserve. If you are to attain and maintain a healthy, fit body, you have to learn to get back in touch with your body. What foods does it want for fuel? What kinds of physical activity make it feel good? Once you ask these questions—and learn to listen to your body's answer—you are halfway there. Learning to listen, however, requires time, practice, and patience.

In terms of achieving a healthy weight, the first "lesson" is to learn the difference between hunger and appetite, and to respond appropriately.

Hunger is a *physiological* state—an internal dinner bell that rings when the body requires fuel (food). The "bell" triggers strong responses: Our stomachs growl, we can't stop thinking about food, and we take action to find it. Hunger pangs are the body's signal to eat. The inner feeling of satisfaction, or *satiety*, is its way of saying, "I've had my fill, thanks."

Appetite, on the other hand, is the *desire*, rather than the need, to eat. Hunger isn't a prerequisite for appetite, as any woman who's scarfed down the two leftover slices of pizza 2 hours after eating can attest. An attractive, tasty meal may tickle our appetites long after our hunger has been satisfied. We eat anyway because, well, we like the taste of pizza, or we're in the company of friends and feeling happy and sociable. Or maybe we eat because we're bored or sad or angry and—because we have pleasant memories of eating—we use the pizza to lift our mood.

Asking your body whether it is asking for food to satisfy physical hunger or a hungry heart—and answering honestly—will slowly alter the way you think about food, making you less likely to overeat. For the first week, before you put fork to mouth, I want you to ask your body these simple questions. Ask the questions in "you" form, as if you were talking to a friend or a child.

ARE YOU ASKING FOR FUEL OR FOR COMFORT? There are several differences between physical and emotional hunger.

❧ Emotional hunger comes on suddenly; physical hunger, gradually.

❧ Emotional hunger triggers a craving for a specific food—pizza, macaroni and cheese, ice cream—and only that food will satisfy it.

❧ Emotional hunger drives you to continue eating long after you're full.

❧ Emotional eating triggers guilt; physical hunger does not.

Take a minute. Close your eyes if you're alone, and really listen: Is your stomach growling to be fed? Or is it your heart that is screaming to eat?

IF THE ANSWER IS FUEL: WHAT DO YOU NEED? Unless you are in the throes of PMS, if the answer is "cookies" or "chips," it's not your body talking. It's your heart. Gently tell your body that the foods it is requesting are not fuel. They're tasty, certainly, but they are not good sources of nutrients and energy. Ask again, and wait. (If you *are* in the throes of PMS, see "What I Eat (and How I Cheat)" on page 265 for my advice.)

IF THE ANSWER IS COMFORT: HOW CAN I HELP? Does your body need a walk around the block to blow off steam, or a workout to discharge anger? Is your body lonely and in need of the companionship of another body? Perhaps it needs a short nap to ease fatigue, which causes stress. It may sound funny at first—talking to your body as if it is a friend. But think about it. If you begin to treat it as kindly as you would a friend, you will not want to harm it with a guilt-inducing eating binge. You will want to encourage its efforts to be fit and healthy.

ARE YOU SATISFIED OR UNCOMFORTABLY STUFFED? After you eat, ask your body that question.

I'll bet these questions took you by surprise. I'll bet you were waiting for me to tell you to keep a food diary. Unlike some fitness experts, I make it an option, not a requirement. Some women find logging their food intake quite helpful, and I encourage you to give it a try if it has helped you in the past, or if you've never kept one before. Other women find that simply asking themselves the questions above each time they wish to eat works just as well. When you think about it, both methods have the same goal: to foster mindful eating.

LEAN-FOR-LIFE PRACTICE:
UPGRADE YOUR CARBOHYDRATES

I ask that you not eliminate any food groups from your diet, carbohydrates included. But I do recommend that you *upgrade* them.

MINNA'S SHOPPING CART

If you caught up with me in the grocery store, here's what you might see in my cart.

❖ **FRUITS AND VEGGIES**—organic, mostly. I love papayas, bananas, strawberries, blueberries, mangoes, watermelon, broccoli (my favorite veggie!), sweet potatoes, peppers, fresh spinach, asparagus, green beans.

❖ **LEAN MEATS AND FISH**—free-range chicken, Chilean sea bass (it's the one fish my one daughter will eat, so we eat it once a week!), salmon, tilapia, deli turkey, the occasional cut of lean red meat (filet mignon, or 96% fat-free ground beef).

❖ **DAIRY**—organic milk, eggs, deli white American cheese, organic low-fat yogurt and cottage cheese, low-fat cheddar, mozzarella, ricotta cheeses, ice cream for my girls and husband (oh, okay, and for me, too).

❖ **WHOLE GRAINS**—old-fashioned oatmeal, Cheerios (my girls love them), brown and whole grain rice, whole grain bread, Hodgson Mill Organic pastas (loaded with fiber and higher protein content), black and red beans (I *love* beans seasoned with cilantro).

"Upgrading" your carbs means trading up. Replace the simple carbohydrates that encourage weight gain, such as cookies, sodas, chips, and most grab-and-go processed foods, with healthier complex carbohydrates—whole grains, beans, fruits, and veggies, all of which curb cravings and help reduce excess body fat. You'll eat hearty, and your body will get the vitamins, minerals, and other substances essential to good health. Chances are that shortly after you "upgrade," your energy and mental alertness will skyrocket because your body will be getting the nutrients it needs for physical and mental labor. You'll probably feel less bloated, too.

Upgrading your carbs is simpler than you think. Here are four easy ways to do it.

✤ Upgrade from white to whole grain bread. Best bets include Pepperidge Farm 100% Stone Ground Whole Wheat Bread, Wonder Stone Ground 100% Whole Wheat Bread, and Thomas's Sahara 100% Whole Wheat Pita Bread. Tried it and don't like it? When you make a sandwich, use your favorite bread on top and whole grain on the bottom. Get fiber-conscious, too. Scout out some of the natural, whole grain breads in health-food stores, opting for varieties that pack 3 to 4 grams or more of fiber per slice.

✤ Upgrade from white rice to whole grains. Brown rice is a start, but poke around your local natural-foods store. You'll find a treasure trove of delicious, nutritious whole grains, including bulgur, barley, buckwheat, spelt, and oats. For more information on these grains and recipes, log on to www.wholegrainscouncil.org.

✤ Upgrade from white flour and sugar to whole grain flours and natural sweeteners. Buy baked goods made with whole grain flours and natural sweeteners, and use these ingredients in your home-baked goods, as well. Replace half of the white flour called for in your regular recipes for cookies, muffins, quick breads, and pancakes with whole wheat flour. Or replace up to 20 percent of white flour with another whole grain flour, such as sorghum. (Of course, if you're trying to lose weight, enjoy a small slice of cake or a fresh-baked muffin once or twice a week.)

✤ Upgrade from white to whole grain pasta. I love chewy, nutty-tasting whole wheat pasta. If you don't, try one of the new "hybrid" pastas that combine 60 percent whole grain flour and refined flour. You'll find them in natural-foods stores and larger supermarkets. And check your local natural-foods store for other whole grain pastas made with brown rice and buckwheat.

MINNA'S CAN'T-GO-WRONG FOOD LIST

Now that I've armed you with what you need to know to achieve a lean, sculpted body, use this handy-dandy food list—complete with serving sizes—to create your own healthy, nutritious meals. Simply combine one serving of lean protein with one serving each of healthy carbohydrate and fat, and you're good to go!

LEAN PROTEINS: EGGS, CHEESE, AND REDUCED-FAT DAIRY

Cheese, light or fat free, 2 oz

Low-fat yogurt, 8 oz

Whole egg, 1

Egg whites, 3 to 4

Egg substitute, ⅓ to ½ cup

Low-fat cottage cheese, ½ cup

Low-fat milk (fat free or 1%), 8 oz

Fat-free ricotta cheese, ⅓ cup

LEAN PROTEINS: FISH (3-OZ SERVING)

Catfish

Haddock

Salmon

Shellfish (shrimp, crab, lobster)

Tuna

LEAN PROTEINS: SOY FOODS

Soy cheese, 2 oz

Soy milk, 8 oz

Soy nuts, ¼ to ⅓ cup

Tofu, 4 oz

LEAN PROTEINS: MEAT OR POULTRY (3-OZ SERVING)

Skinless chicken

Skinless turkey

Lean beef

Lean pork

Lean deli meat

HEALTHY CARBOHYDRATES: FRUITS (1 WHOLE FRUIT OR ½ CUP BERRIES)

Apples

Strawberries, blueberries, raspberries

Oranges and other citrus fruits

HEALTHY CARBOHYDRATES: GRAINS (½-CUP SERVING)

Whole wheat bread, 1 slice

Whole wheat pita or wrap, ½

Steamed brown or wild rice, ½ cup cooked

Whole wheat pasta, ½ cup cooked

Oatmeal, ½ cup cooked

HEALTHY CARBOHYDRATES: VEGETABLES
(½-CUP SERVING)

Artichoke

Asparagus

Beans

Bell pepper

Broccoli

Brussels sprouts

Cabbage

Carrots

Cauliflower

Celery

Cucumber

Green beans

Lettuce

Mushrooms

Onion

Pumpkin

Spinach

Squash

Sweet potato

Tomato

Zucchini

HEALTHY FATS: NUTS AND OILS

Natural peanut butter, 1 tablespoon

Nuts: 15 almonds, 20 peanuts, 12 walnut halves

Olive oil, canola oil, or safflower oil, 1 tablespoon

ELIMINATE OR EAT SPARINGLY

Refined ("white") sugar and white starches, including white pasta

Convenience foods

Processed meats (bologna, hot dogs, sausage)

Full-fat red meat and cheese (high in saturated fat)

Corn, potatoes, and other starchy vegetables

WEEK 2
LEAN-FOR-LIFE PRINCIPLE:
EAT "CLOSE TO NATURE"

Nowadays, sadly, it is challenging to eat fresh and natural foods; it seems that every product on the supermarket shelves is processed and chemically altered. Chemically processed foods interfere with and ultimately damage your body's integrity. Foods in their most natural state preserve it.

If your body is "asking" for diet foods filled with artificial flavors and colors, it's because it has become used to that kind of empty nutrition.

Fake foods disrupt your awareness of what your body is asking for, nutrition-wise. Your body's response is to ask for more of it because it doesn't satisfy. For example, you may eat half a box of low-fat cookies to satisfy your craving for the real thing. Dare I say this practice is "pound foolish"?

You must retrain your body to ask for foods that will maximize your health and fitness. Before you buy a product, read its list of ingredients. If you can't pronounce most of the items listed, it's probably a good idea to pass it up. Also, beware: Companies are getting smarter and smarter about disguising not-so-good ingredients—if something seems too good to be true, it probably is. So if a sweet-tasting product's ingredient list has no sugar and no artificial sweetener that you recognize, there's almost definitely a chemical sweetener hidden among those long names.

I love the national grocery chain Trader Joe's. It offers fresh, organic, and healthy prepared foods at competitive prices. If you're pressed for time—and who isn't?—it also carries quick-and-healthy fare such as burritos, soups, frozen fish, salads, ultra-healthy whole grain breads and muffins, and sandwiches. To find a store near you, log on to www.traderjoes.com.

LEAN-FOR-LIFE PRACTICE:
LEAN UP YOUR PROTEIN

Protein is found throughout the body—from your muscles and bones to your skin and hair. It makes up the enzymes that power many chemical reactions and the hemoglobin that carries oxygen in your blood. At least 10,000 different proteins make you what you are and keep you that way. Approximately 20 basic building blocks, called amino acids, provide the raw material for all proteins. Because the body doesn't store amino acids, as it does fats or carbohydrates, it needs a daily supply of amino acids to make new protein.

If you eat healthfully, you will get enough protein. The key is to choose *lean* protein. That means to consider a protein's "packaging." Some foods "wrap" their protein in unhealthy fat (think prime rib or whole milk). Here's a list of lean protein sources that will deliver the nutrients your body needs without the unhealthy saturated fat that it doesn't.

❖ Without the skin and cooked without fat, chicken and turkey are low in fat and incredibly versatile.

❖ Fish is simple to prepare and serve: Arrange your favorite veggies in a baking dish and drizzle them with oil. Roast or steam them until almost tender, then add your favorite fillet to the dish. In minutes, you'll have perfectly cooked fish and sumptuous vegetables on the side. *Note:* Due to high mercury levels, the FDA recommends that women who are pregnant or of childbearing age and children under the age of 5 limit their consumption of shrimp, salmon, pollack, catfish, and "light" canned tuna to no more than twice a week and albacore tuna—also called "solid white" or "chunk white" tuna—to no more than once a week. Haddock, wild Pacific salmon, and farmed catfish or trout are excellent low-mercury choices. Pregnant women should also avoid consuming raw fish to reduce their risk of exposure to parasites and germs.

❖ Low-fat cottage cheese contains all the amino acids necessary to build new muscle.

❖ Soy foods, such as tofu and soy milk, are excellent sources of low-fat, nutrient-dense protein. Add tofu to chili, eggs, or casseroles—you'll never taste it because it absorbs the flavor of whatever you're cooking it with. Use soy milk in place of whole milk on cereal and in baked goods, or use it as a base for a tasty fruit smoothie.

❖ Eggs contain a variety of important nutrients. If you are watching your cholesterol, opt for using just egg whites. Low in calories, with zero cholesterol and fat, egg whites cook up into delicious, fluffy scrambled eggs and omelets.

❖ Beans, nuts, and whole grains offer plenty of healthful fiber and micronutrients with a minimum of saturated fat.

✤ Red meat is an excellent source of protein—if you opt for the leanest cuts. Whenever possible, choose "select," the leanest grade of beef, found in cuts such as eye of round, top round, and top sirloin.

✤ If you like dairy products, skim milk, reduced-fat cheeses, and low-fat yogurt are the healthiest choices.

SLOW DOWN, YOU EAT TOO FAST

I first became aware of the benefits of eating slowly in college. I was training for an aerobic competition and had heard that eating slowly helps you eat less, so I thought I'd give it a try.

I'd already switched to eating smaller, more frequent meals. Pacing myself was a bit trickier. Still, I chewed slowly. I made myself put down my fork between bites. If I had a dining companion, I talked more, so I didn't automatically reach for seconds. If I was eating alone, I read a book.

After a few weeks, this unhurried pace felt "right." I felt lighter and—far from feeling starved—had energy to burn. My metabolism revved up, too: Like clockwork, my body asked for food every 2 to 3 hours, I fed it another small meal, it asked for food again in another few hours, I fed it another mini-meal.

Eating slowly doesn't work just for me. In fact, one recent study found that eating slowly for the first 10 minutes of a meal may turn off the brain's "appetite switch," helping you to eat less and pare away the pounds. So if you can pace yourself for 10 minutes, you'll likely be satisfied with a smaller meal. If you're still a bit hungry after you eat, do something to take your mind off food for at least 20 minutes—take a brisk walk, polish your toenails, do some weeding in the garden. Your hunger will most likely subside—*if* you listened to your body and fed it what it asked for.

I ate slowly until I became a mom. (Who ever heard of a small child willing to sit at the table for more than 10 minutes?) Eating quickly feels uncomfortable to me now, and I notice that I don't enjoy my meals as much. There's no time to savor the flavor, enjoy the experience.

However, sometimes these rush-rush meals work to my advantage because I get to eat only about a third of my meal. When my littlest one stands up in her high chair and cries to be on my lap, it can take me a very long time to eat!

WEEK 3
LEAN-FOR-LIFE PRINCIPLE:
EAT LESS, MORE OFTEN

Your mother probably told you to eat three square meals a day. But if you're trying to lose weight, that may be bad advice. To keep your metabolism going strong, ditch the usual three big meals and eat six smaller ones of about 250 calories each throughout the day.

Studies suggest that eating smaller amounts more frequently—every 3 hours or so—is the way to go. In one such study, researchers at the University of Massachusetts in Worcester found that people who ate four or more times daily—generally three "mini-meals" and one or two snacks—were less likely to be overweight than were those who ate fewer, larger meals.

If you usually skip meals or starve yourself to lose weight, eating every few hours may seem like an unlikely way to save calories—until you consider that big, infrequent meals actually *slow* your metabolism. It's true. When you starve yourself, the body senses that food is scarce and conserves its reserves, slowing its metabolism to hold on to what it has until the next big meal comes along.

If you are used to eating big meals spaced far apart, it make take some adjusting to get used to eating less at one sitting. Remind yourself that you will be eating again soon—sooner than you used to! Also, pay attention to how much better you feel after a smaller meal. You have satisfied your hunger rather than stuffed yourself to the point of discomfort.

MINNA'S NUTRITION PRINCIPLES AND PRACTICE

Week 1

❖ LEAN-FOR-LIFE PRINCIPLE: Learn the difference between hunger and appetite.

❖ LEAN-FOR-LIFE PRACTICE: Upgrade your carbohydrates.

Week 2

❖ LEAN-FOR-LIFE PRINCIPLE: Eat "close to nature."

❖ LEAN-FOR-LIFE PRACTICE: Lean up your protein.

Week 3

❖ LEAN-FOR-LIFE PRINCIPLE: Eat less, more often.

❖ LEAN-FOR-LIFE PRACTICE: Water yourself daily.

Week 4

❖ LEAN-FOR-LIFE PRINCIPLE: Don't be a slave to your scale.

❖ LEAN-FOR-LIFE PRACTICE: Don't skimp on healthy fats.

Here are a few examples of healthy mini-meals.

BREAKFAST
* 2 or 3 scrambled egg whites, ¼ cup of whole grain oatmeal
* 1 small container of low-fat yogurt topped with slivered almonds and orange segments
* 1 slice of whole wheat toast, 1 scrambled egg, 2 slices of turkey bacon

LUNCH
* 1 turkey breast sandwich on whole wheat bread with lettuce and tomato, 1 banana
* 1 can of light tuna mixed with balsamic dressing, 3 to 5 whole grain crackers, 1 small piece of fruit

DINNER
* 3 ounces of lean grilled chicken, ½ cup of steamed brown rice, a small green salad dressed with vinegar and olive oil
* 1 serving (3 to 4 ounces) of lean red meat or poultry, or 1 cup of whole grain pasta tossed with zucchini, yellow squash, bell peppers, tomatoes, and 1 teaspoon of grated Parmesan cheese

SNACKS
* 1 frozen fruit bar
* 1 ready-to-eat cereal bar, such as Nutri-Grain brand, warmed in the microwave for less than a minute and then spread with 1 teaspoon of low-fat cream cheese
* 1 whole wheat tortilla, 1 slice of avocado, 2 slices of chicken breast, tomato, lettuce, and 1 tablespoon of salsa
* ½ whole wheat English muffin, 1 ounce of reduced-fat mozzarella cheese, and tomato slices
* 1 small package of precut veggies with reduced-fat dip

LEAN-FOR-LIFE PRACTICE:
WATER YOURSELF DAILY

When I wake up in the morning, one of the first things I do is down a tall glass of water. I also "water myself" throughout the day. Drinking lots of water while you're switching over to a healthy way of eating can help you shed those extra pounds, but not because the water fills you up or flushes toxins out of your system. The real reason is that water tends to squelch food cravings. Lots of people think they're hungry when they really need something to drink. As a result, they eat to satisfy their thirst. Next time you have what you think is a craving for food, try sipping a small amount of water. If it's fluid your body is "hungering" for, you may be able to resist those midafternoon or nighttime munchies.

The key to quenching cravings with water isn't how much of it you drink but how frequently. Small amounts sipped at frequent intervals work better than a full glass gulped down like medicine. These tips can help you meet your water quota of eight 8-ounce glasses per day.

✤ Drink up before breakfast. Your body can really use a long, cool drink after a long, dry night.

✤ Have a glass of water whenever you have a snack.

✤ Keep a refillable water bottle handy in the fridge and get in the habit of grabbing it on your way out the door.

WEEK 4
LEAN-FOR-LIFE PRINCIPLE:
DON'T BE A SLAVE TO YOUR SCALE

Do you hop on the scale more than once a day? If so, chances are good that you feel defeated when the number doesn't budge—or frustrated if it goes up a pound or two. That's why I tell my clients to weigh themselves no more than twice per month— every other week.

I practice what I preach. I step on the scale once a year—at my annual physical exam. I couldn't care less what the scale says. It's about how I feel in my body. If I don't feel good, I make the necessary changes to feel good again. For example, maybe I've neglected my abs lately and I notice I feel uncomfortable in that area—maybe my belly is protruding a bit. So I tighten my diet and increase the intensity of my workouts a little. I do not get on the scale every day to see if I've lost a pound. Weight is dynamic, and it reacts to changes in hormones, water intake, and a variety of other factors.

Some women lose a pound on Tuesday and regain it on Wednesday, and this 1 measly pound makes or breaks them mentally and emotionally. I can still hear some of my clients, early on in their training, their voices full of defeat: "I gained 2 pounds today! I don't understand. I'm working so hard and I gain weight? I may as well not work out at all!"

One of my clients had a love/hate relationship with her scale. When her scale said she'd lost 2 pounds, she'd rush to the gym high as a kite, and her workout reflected her excitement. We'd make real progress, because her motivation and drive were in total unison.

At the next workout she'd drag herself in, head down, shoulders drooping. "Don't tell me," I'd say. "You gained a pound." She'd nod glumly. On those days, her workouts suffered. It was like pulling teeth to get her to finish a set.

Finally, after much coaxing, I convinced her to "break up" with her scale. (Her husband actually locked it up!) For 3 months, I took her measurements instead. The relief was immediate, but after 3 weeks, she started to get really excited. For the first time, she really felt her results instead of merely seeing them on a scale. We kept going with it; at each workout, her mood was good and her efforts were consistent. After 2 months, she was able to slip into an old jogging outfit she'd worn in college! By the end of 3 months, she was shopping for new clothing. She felt like a new woman—attitude over all.

When her scaleless 90 days were up, I said, "Okay. Jump on." She had lost 27 pounds.

I jumped for joy, screamed, cheered—I must have looked crazy to anyone who passed by. She stood there with a faint smile on her face and said, "Minna, it's just a number." I stopped dead—was this the same woman I'd met 6 months before? Then she burst out laughing—and crying—as she thanked me for freeing her from her scale. (For all I know, it's still locked up!)

I urge you to shed your scale, too. If you want evidence of your progress, measure your neck, bust, waist, hips, biceps, upper thighs, and calves every 2 weeks, always in the same spot. Follow my workout and eating plan faithfully, and you too could be as pleasantly surprised as my client was.

LEAN-FOR-LIFE PRACTICE:
DON'T SKIMP ON HEALTHY FATS

Fats and oils are part of a healthful diet. They supply your body with energy and essential fatty acids, help it absorb fat-soluble vitamins, and play a key role in countless body functions.

Dietary fat is found in foods of both plant and animal origin. It's the type and amount of fat you eat that makes a difference. High intakes of saturated fats trans fats, and cholesterol increase the risk of unhealthy blood lipid levels, which in turn may increase the risk of coronary heart disease. Other chronic health problems, such as obesity, may be caused or worsened by high-fat diets.

Saturated fat and trans fats (fats that are solid at room temperature) appear to carry the greatest amount of risk. To lower your intake of saturated fat, limit your intake of animal fats found in foods such as butter, ice cream, bacon, sausage, and other fatty meats.

By looking at the food label, you can select the products that are lowest in saturated and trans fats. Eating fewer processed foods is the most effective way to reduce your intake of trans fats. Trans fats are listed in the food ingredient list on product packaging as "partially hydrogenated" oils and are quantified on the nutrition facts label.

Some fats, such as canola and olive oil, are healthier choices than others. These fats are liquid at room temperature. Fish are an excellent source of omega-3 fatty acids, which have been found to foster good health.

APPENDIX

TRAINING LOGS

TANK TOP ARMS

DATE:	DURATION OF WORKOUT:

CARDIO/NOTES:

IN THE "MOVE" BOX, WRITE EACH MOVE PERFORMED.
IN THE FIRST HALF OF THE "SET" BOX, RECORD THE AMOUNT OF WEIGHT YOU LIFTED.
IN THE OTHER HALF, RECORD THE NUMBER OF REPETITIONS COMPLETED.

MOVE	SET 1 WEIGHT / REPS	SET 2 WEIGHT / REPS	SET 3 WEIGHT / REPS

BIKINI BELLY

DATE:	DURATION OF WORKOUT:

CARDIO/NOTES:

IN THE "MOVE" BOX, WRITE EACH MOVE PERFORMED.
IN THE FIRST HALF OF THE "SET" BOX, RECORD THE AMOUNT OF WEIGHT YOU LIFTED.
IN THE OTHER HALF, RECORD THE NUMBER OF REPETITIONS COMPLETED.

MOVE	SET 1		SET 2		SET 3	
	WEIGHT	REPS	WEIGHT	REPS	WEIGHT	REPS

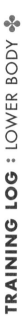

BOY SHORTS BOTTOM

DATE:	DURATION OF WORKOUT:

CARDIO/NOTES:

IN THE "MOVE" BOX, WRITE EACH MOVE PERFORMED.
IN THE FIRST HALF OF THE "SET" BOX, RECORD THE AMOUNT OF WEIGHT YOU LIFTED.
IN THE OTHER HALF, RECORD THE NUMBER OF REPETITIONS COMPLETED.

MOVE	SET 1		SET 2		SET 3	
	WEIGHT	REPS	WEIGHT	REPS	WEIGHT	REPS

❖

INDEX

Boldface page references indicate photographs.

Underscored references indicate boxed text.

Flexibility. *See also* Stretches
   cooldown routines, 48–49
   factors influencing, 45
   importance of training, 19, 20
   loss of, 20
   moving, 20–21
   static stretching, 20–21
   stretching safely, 45–46
   warmup
      sports-style, 46–47
      yoga-style, 47–48
Flour, 269
Fly
   chest, 86–87, **87**
   rear deltoid, 74–75, **75**
Food
   to avoid, 271
   eating slowly, 274
   ingredients list, 272
   list, author's, 270–71
   meals
      healthy mini-meals, 276
      size and frequency, 275
   menu, author's, 265
   natural, 272
   postworkout, 240
   shopping cart, author's, 268
Form, focus on, 213
Frequency, of cardio workouts, 8
Froggy double-leg lift, 188, **188**
Front raise, 54, **55**
Front to side plank, 96–97, **97**
Fruits, 270
Functional training
   benefits, 3–4
   strength training compared, 2–3
Funky abs, 118–19, **119**

❖G

Gender, influence on flexibility, 45
Goals, setting, 222–23
Grains, whole, 270, 273
Gymnast abs, 152–53, **153**

❖H

Hammer curl, 64–65, **65**
Heart rate
   maximum (MHR), 8–9
   monitoring by Talk Test, 10
   target (THR), 8–10
Heart-rate monitor, 10
Hip extension, 170, **171**
   standing, 194–95, **195**
Hunger
   appetite differentiated from, 266–67
   physical and emotional, 267
   taking edge off, 240
Hurdler, modified, 27, **27**

❖I

Intensity
   high-intensity zone, 9–10
   interval training, 11, 13–14
   low-intensity zone, 9
   maximum heart rate (MHR), 8–9
   moderate-intensity zone, 9
   physical activities defined by level of, 12
   rate of perceived exertion (RPE), 10–11
   target heart rate (THR), 8–10
Interval training, 11, 13–14

❖J

Joint integrity, 3

❖K

Knee drop, 158–59, **159**
Knee/heel tap, 176–77, **177**
Kneeling lunge, 25, **25,** 35, **35**

❖L

Lateral raise, 72–73, **73**
Leg abduction, 178–79, **179**
Leg extension, 154, **155**
Leg lift, 174–75, **175**
   double, 112, **113**
   froggy double, 188, **188**
   reverse plank with, 206, **207**

Snacks
  after-workout, <u>240</u>
  healthy examples, 276
Soreness, muscle, 213
Soy foods, 270, 273
Spinal twist, 31, **31**
Split-leg lunge, 202–3, **203**
Split leg stretch, 34, **34**
Sports-style warmup, 46–47
Squat, 166–67, **167**
  one-legged, 204–5, **205**
  plié, 192, **193**
Standing hip extension, 194–95, **195**
Standing quadriceps stretch, 28, **28**
Static stretching, 20–21. *See also* Stretches,
  static
Stationary lunge, 180–81, **181**
Step-up, 168–69, **169**
Stress busters, <u>223</u>
Stretches
  moving flexibility
    bent-arm overhead, 38, **38**
    chair to standing forward bend, 33, **33**
    child's pose with reach across, 42, **42**
    child's pose with upward-facing dog, 44,
      44
    kneeling lunge, 35, **35**
    lunge with one-arm reach, 43, **43**
    lying leg split, 36, **36**
    open arm, 41, **41**
    single-arm reach across, 37, **37**
    single-arm reach back, 39, **39**
    split leg, 34, **34**
    walking quadriceps, 40, **40**
  safety guidelines, 45–46
  static
    child's pose with reach across, 30,
      30
    cobra pose, 32, **32**
    kneeling lunge, 25, **25**
    modified hurdler, 27, **27**
    one-arm round front, 29, **29**
    reaching butterfly, 24, **24**

    seated forward bend, 23, **23**
    single-arm reach across, 26, **26**
    spinal twist, 31, **31**
    standing quadriceps, 28, **28**
  use before, during, and after workout,
    22
Sugar, 269
Superman, 134–35, **135**
Sweetener, natural, 269

♣T

Talk Test, 10
Tank Top Arms
  Master exercises
    Arnold press, 102–3, **103**
    bent-over row, 98–99, **99**
    front to side plank, 96–97, **97**
    one-arm triceps pushup, 94–95, **95**
    plank hold walkout, 90–91, **91**
    shoulder shimmy, 104–5, **105**
    side plank with arm raise, 100–101, **101**
    yogi pushup, 92, **93**
  Novice exercises
    biceps curl, 62–63, **63**
    chest press, 66–67, **67**
    front raise, 54, **55**
    hammer curl, 64–65, **65**
    lying triceps extension, 60, **61**
    modified pushup, 68, **69**
    shoulder press, 56, **57**
    triceps kickback, 58, **59**
  Skilled exercises
    chest fly, 86–87, **87**
    concentration curl, 84–85, **85**
    lateral raise, 72–73, **73**
    modified plank, 76–77, **77**
    overhead triceps extension, 78, **79**
    rear deltoid fly, 74–75, **75**
    rotational shoulder press, 82, **82**
    triceps dip, 80, **80**
  training log, 282
Target heart rate (THR), 8–10
Temperature, influence on flexibility, 45

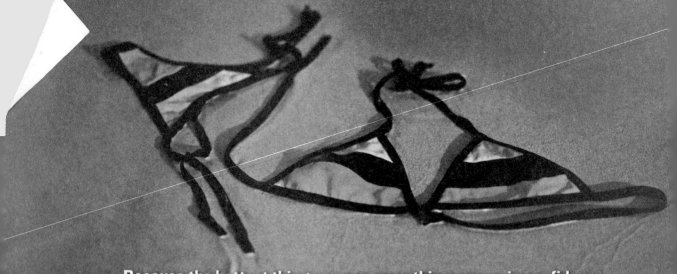

Because the hottest thing you can wear this summer is confidence.

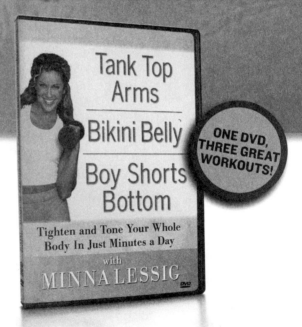

Tank Top Arms

Bikini Belly

Boy Shorts Bottom

Tighten and Tone Your Whole Body In Just Minutes a Day

with

MINNA LESSIG

ONE DVD, THREE GREAT WORKOUTS!

The **TANK TOP ARMS, BIKINI BELLY, BOY SHORTS BOTTOM** DVD workout will forever change the way you look, feel, and think about your body. This 60-minute workout is comprised of three segments, each targeting one of the most common trouble spots women face. Shape jiggle-proof arms, a flatter, sexier stomach, and a firm backside by the time summer arrives. Internationally recognized fitness trainer Minna Lessig instructs you to help you achieve proper form for every move and to make sure your body gets more out of every minute.

AVAILABLE WHEREVER DVDs ARE SOLD.

ORDER YOURS NOW AT: (800) 266-9719 OR WWW.TANKTOPARMSBIKINIBELLY.COM

RODALE

LIVE YOUR WHOLE LIFE